Tufts University Friedman School of Nutrition Science and Policy
Produced in conjunction with Castaway Media
Cover photo by Lisa D. Fryxell

Tufts Media LLC
196 Boston Ave., Suite 2100
Medford, MA 02155 USA

The Best in Health & Nutrition 2007
The year's most important news for living healthier longer.
The editors of the Tufts University Health & Nutrition Letter

ISBN: 978-0-9765728-4-8
1. Health   2. Nutrition

Library of Congress Control Number: 2007920158

Manufactured in the United States of America

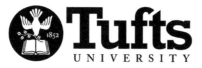

Friedman School of Nutrition Science and Policy
Eileen Kennedy, DSc, Dean

The Best in Health & Nutrition 2007

*The year's most important news
for living healthier longer.*

Scientific Editor: Irwin H. Rosenberg, MD,
University Professor, Tufts University

Managing Editor: David A. Fryxell

Based on a full year's content of the *Tufts University Health & Nutrition Letter*—
updated, organized and fully indexed for easy reference.

Table of Contents

Osteoarthritis • Vitamin D Drives Bone Health—and You May Not Be Getting Enough • Even Moderate Exercise Staves Off Arthritis Decline • New Twist on Back Pain Treatment—Yoga • Calcium, Vitamin D and Bone Health: Now What Should You Do? • Bone Testing Missing Those Most at Risk

The Sour Truth About Apple-Cider Vinegar • The Minuses of
Juice Plus • Does Chromium Shine vs. Diabetes? • Canola Oil
Fears • Weighing Iron Supplementation • Pectin Against Cancer?
• How Much Folate? • Focus on Eye-Supplement Overlap •
Blood Type Diet

Message from the Dean

In academia, and particularly in Boston, a 25-year-old school is relatively "young" among its partners in higher education. So as we celebrate our first quarter-century, the accomplishments of taking our educational mandate beyond the Boston campus are worthy of note. These accomplishments, and the many that have preceded them, have helped make our "young" school a world leader in nutrition science and policy.

The 2006-07 academic year will have three significant "firsts," each of which take the Friedman School's application of nutrition science and policy to students and professionals beyond our borders.

In September, we hosted the inaugural Friedman School Symposium, a two-and-a-half-day conference with a focus on some of the key issues that will become part of the USDA's 2010 revision of the Dietary Guidelines for Americans.

Highlights of the symposium included:

• Bringing scientists, practitioners, policymakers and food industry representatives together for open dialogue on key issues that affect the health of US and world citizens.

• Attracting 27 of the world's foremost researchers and policy influencers—each of whom gave leading-edge presentations on topics as diverse as genetics, micronutrients, obesity, hydration, probiotics, communications and corporate roles in nutrition.

• Bringing our own students together with professionals in a variety of careers to exchange ideas and learn about careers in nutrition.

I was particularly delighted to find that our students were eager to participate (more than 40 students applied for and received scholarships to attend the sessions) and become part of the dialogue. Friedman School students also submitted posters featuring their research for display at a poster session. Eight research projects from seven of our students were displayed at the symposium. Congratulations to our poster session participants.

By the numbers, we had just over 250 attendees at our first conference. They came from eight countries, including Taiwan, Mexico and Peru. Sixteen universities from across the country and around the world were represented, and we received educational grants from 25 organizations, most representing the food industry, but also including the federal government (NIH Office of Dietary Supplements) and one international organization, the International Union of Nutrition Science.

The symposium has reinforced the Friedman School's leadership in bringing all stakeholders in nutrition together to learn about the most recent science and policy advances. Our second symposium will take place in the fall of 2007 and promises to attract an even broader audience by continuing the practice of bringing the best presenters on their individual subjects to the Friedman School.

Another "first" for the Friedman School is the student-run Day of Research conference, which will take place in March 2007. Led entirely by a team of students, this event will bring graduate students in nutrition-related fields from Tufts and other leading universities together for a full day of research presentations. Panel discussions, poster presentations and roundtable sessions will give students the opportunity to refine their presentation skills, learn from their peers and network with fellow future leaders from the visiting universities. This event is intended to become an annual gathering of the region's top students.

Finally, you are holding the "first" ever annual book based on the content of the award-winning *Tufts University Health & Nutrition Letter,* which takes our educational mandate beyond Boston to a national audience of readers looking for the best research and advice on health and nutrition.

I am especially pleased to bring you this book, and truly hope that it helps each of you live a healthier life, longer.

Eileen Kennedy, DSc.
Dean, Friedman School of Nutrition Science and Policy
Tufts University

Understanding Nutrition Research Studies

Studying Research Studies: 10 Questions You Need to Ask

A wire story in your local newspaper reports that a new study says flavonoids—antioxidants found in plants, tea, coffee and even chocolate—reduce postmenopausal women's risk of breast cancer by 45%. This sounds like great news—an easy, even enjoyable way to ward off one of the diseases women fear most. But before you load up in the produce aisle, brew an extra pot of tea or coffee and give yourself an excuse to gobble a candy bar, read beyond the headlines.

Understanding what research studies really mean can keep you from bouncing from one health fad to another—and from feeling disappointed, confused and even betrayed when a newer study seems to contradict the research around which you've just reorganized your diet and lifestyle. Learning to read between the lines of research reports can also keep you from missing significant findings that might benefit your health.

"Consumers figure that the silly scientists have just changed their minds again. So why bother listening to the next piece of nutrition advice at all?" is how Dayle Hayes, MS, RD, a registered dietician and consultant to Deaconess Billings Clinic in Montana, describes the dilemma. "In fact, any one study is just one piece of a large research puzzle. Research into any topic is always a work in progress."

That means taking any single study with a grain of salt—and some with a whole shaker. Take that flavonoids study, which was reported by media ranging from the *New York Times* News Service to *Forbes* to the DrKoop.com Web site.

"I'm flabbergasted that reputable news services would pick that up," says Alice H. Lichtenstein, DSc, senior scientist and director of the

Cardiovascular Nutrition Laboratory at Tufts' Jean Mayer USDA Human Nutrition Research Center on Aging. Lichtenstein, who is frequently quoted in news reports about recent research findings, adds, "There is a bias in reporting positive results by the press. Smaller studies at the beginning of rigorously testing a hypothesis get too much attention, while negative studies don't get as many headlines. So everybody gets excessively revved up, and frequently let down in the end.

"People more readily latch onto easy answers—like 'chocolate is really good for me'—than harder things like, 'Weight loss is really important,'" she continues. "Everyone likes to see great results—I'm not against good news. But there are so many examples of good news fizzling."

So flavonoids may someday prove to help prevent breast cancer; a quick check of the PubMed Web site <www. pubmed.gov>, from the National Library of Medicine and the National Institutes of Health (NIH), turns up 667 different studies relating to both flavonoids and breast cancer. But this one new study isn't likely to be the definitive word, Lichtenstein cautions.

1. What type of study?

Why not? For one thing, Lichtenstein points out, the news stories were based on a presentation at the American Association for Cancer Research's annual meeting—not on publication in a **peer-reviewed** scientific journal. Rigorous review by experts in the field—before results are made public—helps put findings in the context of the whole available literature and separate the scientific wheat from the chaff. Publication also gives study authors the opportunity to include any caveats.

Moreover, the study was a **retrospective** one, looking backward in time (in this case, at data from a 1996-97 study). Hayes says, "The usefulness of retrospective research is limited because many factors cannot be controlled, previous data may not have been recorded accurately, and people do not always remember exactly what they did in the past." How much flavonoids did the women *really* consume? A **prospective** study, which follows subjects going forward in time, is generally viewed as more meaningful. So researchers might track women's flavonoid intake over several years, for example, then compare breast-cancer rates between those with the highest and lowest intake.

Both retrospective and prospective studies are types of **observational** studies (also known as **epidemiological** or **population** studies). These look at subjects' health and lifestyle practices but do not intervene—by, say, giving half the women extra flavonoids. "Observational studies can only show associations—they do not show causation," Lichtenstein emphasizes. "They're very good for raising research questions, but the actual associations can only be learned by further research."

By way of example, she points to observational studies that suggested an association between vitamin E supplement use and reduced risk of heart disease and other ailments. Naturally, she says, these appealing results got plenty of press: "It's easy, cheap and you don't have to do anything you don't want to do—just take a pill." Unfortunately, however, followup "intervention" trials (see below) dashed these hopes. That doesn't mean the original observational studies were wrong, Lichtenstein says; perhaps some other "co-association" with the use of vitamin E supplements that led to the observations are important.

To test the associations raised by observational studies, researchers must turn to **clinical trials** (also known as **intervention** studies). The "gold standard" of research studies is the **randomized, controlled, double-blinded trial**. That means the researchers randomly divide participants between study groups, with one group as a control, used as a basis of comparison. Typically, a control group receives a **placebo**—something that looks and tastes like what's being tested—so they don't know which treatment they're getting (a **single-blinded trial**). If neither the participants nor the researchers knows which group is which, to avoid any possible bias, that's a double-blinded trial.

Nine More Questions

Besides looking at what kind of study is making the headlines, what other questions should an informed health consumer ask?

2. Where was it published? Beyond demanding that studies undergo the peer-review process of scholarly publishing, consider where a study does get published. Not all scientific journals carry equal weight. "This is not an absolute," Lichtenstein says, "but generally the better studies tend to be published in the better journals." Besides well-known journals such as the *Journal of the American Medical Association* and *New England Journal of Medicine*, publications to trust include the leading journals in their respective fields, such as those published by the American Heart Association, for example, in cardiovascular research (*Circulation; Hypertension; Circulation Research; Atherosclerosis, Thrombosis and Vascular Biology;* and *Stroke*). In nutrition, respected journals include *The American Journal of Clinical Nutrition* and *The Journal of Nutrition*.

3. Who funded the research? Says Hayes, "Studies funded by a company or an industry are not necessarily biased or inaccurate. The key is to make certain that the study acknowledges its funding source and that it was done as independently as possible." Similarly, be aware that studies paid for by nonprofit groups can be done to promote a particular agenda.

4. Who conducted the research? Lesser-known institutions you've never heard of can still produce groundbreaking research, but you should give greater weight to studies from reputable universities or health centers with a track record for research in this field.

More Terms to Know

Absolute risk–The actual number of health problems that happened or are prevented because of what's being tested: "X number of additional cases in 10,000 people," for example.

Relative risk–A percentage comparing the risk among those in a test group against a control group. A relative risk of 0.7 in a heart-treatment test group means that they were only 70% as likely to suffer heart problems as the placebo group.

Case-Control–A retrospective observational study in which researchers compare two groups–one with the condition being studied (the "case") and one without (the "control")–looking for differences, such as diet or lifestyle.

Cohort–A forward-looking observational study in which a group of people–the cohort–is divided into two or more groups and then followed over a period of time.

Correlation–A statistical association between two or more factors, which does not show cause-and-effect.

Meta-Analysis–A study of studies, collectively analyzing a group of studies on the same subject.

Protocol–The action plan for a clinical trial: what will be done, how it will be conducted, why each step is necessary. Every research center in a multi-location study must follow the same protocol.

---

5. Was it a human trial? Remember that scientists also perform tests using animals or at the cellular level. Results from animal experiments or microscopic studies can help advance scientific frontiers, but you should be cautious about applying these findings to your daily diet.

6. How long did the study last? This isn't as absolute a barometer as you might think: A seven-year study isn't necessarily seven times better than a one-year study. The key, Lichtenstein explains, is whether the study was long enough to adequately measure its desired outcome. A study on fighting cholesterol might require only a month or two, because cholesterol changes relatively quickly. Weight loss takes longer to test: That's why one "low-carb" diet study showed positive results after six months, but after a full year the test and control groups had converged to be little different. Studies of slow-developing diseases might take many years; even a decade might not be enough.

7. How many participants were studied? Again, sheer numbers aren't the slam dunk you might expect. Though an observational study of 50,000 people obviously carries more weight than one of 100 subjects, small numbers can produce meaningful results in clinical trials. The key is whether the study included enough subjects to be **statistically significant**. "You have to look at the study's design," says Lichtenstein. A nutrition study in which just 25 people rotate through four different randomized phases, testing different diets in each—for effects on blood cholesterol, for example—actually carries more statistical weight than a study of 100 people broken into four groups, each trying only one regimen.

8. What kinds of people were included? Were the study participants similar to you in age, gender and other demographic factors, as well as in health condition? Studies looking only at men may—or may not—apply likewise to women. Research on heart-attack or hypertensive subjects may or may not be as applicable to people in general. Populations such as these are frequently studied because it is more likely, if an effect were to occur, that it would be observed in such subjects in a reasonable period of time. But these "secondary prevention" results may not pertain to healthy people ("primary prevention").

9. What do other experts say? The journal may also run an accompanying editorial, commenting on the research. In addition, professional associations such as the American Dietetic Association <www.eatright.org> can help filter the blizzard of research reports, as can national health groups such as the American Cancer Society <www.cancer.org>, American Diabetes Association <www.diabetes.org>, American Heart Association <www.americanheart.org> or the Arthritis Foundation <www.arthritis.org>.

10. What phase was the study? Research on new drug treatments goes through three or four phases. Focus on Phase III trials or later.

Don't rely on these questions alone, however. "The bottom line is—talk to your doctor," concludes a tipsheet from the National Institute on Aging (NIA). "He or she can help you understand the results and what they could mean for your health." Remember, the NIA adds, that medical research progress may take many years: "Every step along the research path provides a clue to the final answer—and probably sparks some new questions also."

To learn more: National Cancer Institute Clinical Trials Factsheet
<www.cancer.gov/cancertopics/factsheet/Information/clinical-trials>.
"Understanding Risk" from the National Institute on Aging
<www.niapublications.org/tipsheets/risk.asp>.

Medical-Meeting News Lost in Media Translation

Not so fast! That's the word from two researchers with the VA Outcomes research group in White River Junction, Vermont, when it comes to media reports out of major medical meetings. Their study concluded that such newspaper and broadcast stories are so often overstated or lacking in basic information and context as to be worthless—or even worse, dangerously misleading.

Steven Woloshin, MD, MS, and Lisa M. Schwartz, MD, MS, both associate professors of medicine at Dartmouth Medical School, reviewed 174 newspaper articles, 32 of which were front-page news stories, as well as 13 radio and television news stories. The news pieces were based on research reported at five scientific meetings, held in 2002 and 2003, of the American Heart Association, the Annual International AIDS Conference, the American Society of Clinical Oncology, the Society for Neuroscience and the Radiological Society of North America.

Their analysis, published in the *Medical Journal of Australia*, found:

• 34% of the stories did not mention how many people or animals were studied

• 18% did not mention study design; another 35% had descriptions so ambiguous that reviewers had to guess

• 40% did not quantify the main result

• 94% of reports about animal studies did not mention that the results might not be applicable to humans

• 90% of stories about uncontrolled studies failed to point out that it was impossible to conclude that the intervention (or treatment) caused the results.

Only two of the news articles about the 175 unpublished studies noted that the findings were not published, might not have been peer-reviewed, and could change before publication. In fact, prior work has shown that 25% of meeting reports garnering media coverage—including page-one stories—are never ultimately published in the medical literature.

Woloshin and Schwartz wrote that research "presented at scientific meetings is generally not ready for public consumption: results change, fatal problems emerge, and the hypotheses fail to pan out."

Their analysis followed a study published in March in *Mayo Clinic Proceedings* that concluded one in five newspaper articles about neurological disorders was wrong. In the Mayo Clinic study, researchers said the media could negatively influence the public's health-related beliefs and behaviors by reporting disproportionately on obscure illnesses with headline appeal and inflaming fears.

In this new report, the Dartmouth experts concluded that since it is unlikely that there will be less reporting at medical meetings in the future, better preparation of materials for the press could aid in accurate and more balanced reporting. To the public, they encouraged a healthy dose of skepticism, stating in their conclusion that "ignoring a preliminary report about a weak study is preferable to being misled."

To learn more: *Medical Journal of Australia,* June 5, 2006; report online at <www.mja.com.au/public/issues/184_11_050606/wol10024_fm.pdf>. *Mayo Clinic Proceedings,* March 2006; abstract at <www.mayoclinicproceedings.com/ Abstract.asp?AID=1659&Abst=Abstract&UID=>.

From the Supermarket to Your Table

Nutrients Report Card Shows Some Failing Grades

If you're a typical American eater, you're probably getting plenty of carbo-hydrates, but not enough vitamin A, C and E and magnesium. And you're still getting too much salt.

Those are among the headlines from the latest snapshot of Americans' dietary habits, based on the ongoing National Health and Nutrition Examination Survey (NHANES), "What We Eat in America." (The report did not measure vitamin D intake, though other studies have found that Americans don't get enough D, either.) The report from the US Department of Agriculture's Agricultural Research Service analyzes NHANES data compiled in 2001-02. To gather the data, 8,940 people answered a question-naire about what they'd eaten in the previous 24 hours; the questionnaire didn't cover vitamin supplements or over-the-counter medications. Follow-up phone interviews filled in any gaps.

The new report compared those responses to the Dietary Reference Intakes for nutrients and dietary components established by the Institute of Medicine.

Besides carbohydrates, the report found that most of us are getting our daily values of selenium, niacin and riboflavin. Children and males general-ly had adequate intakes of protein, folate, copper, phosphorus, thiamin and iron; the proportion of females getting enough of these nutrients was lower, however.

Where are we falling short on nutrients? The report says 93% of Americans aren't getting the recommended daily amount of vitamin E. Slightly more than half fall short on magnesium intake, 44% on vitamin A, about a third on vitamin C.

Some shortfalls were seen only in certain segments of the population. Several groups—older males and older females, plus teenage girls—fail to consume enough zinc. Older women, according to the study, aren't getting enough vitamin B6. Preteen and teenage girls fall short on phosphorus intake.

The report also raised a red flag about low intakes of a number of nutrients for which no Estimated Average Requirements have been established: vitamin K, calcium, potassium and dietary fiber.

What can you do to make sure you're getting adequate amounts of key nutrients? Don't interpret the report as an invitation to start popping vitamin pills. In a recent article in the *Journal of the American Medical Association*, Alice Lichtenstein, DSc, and Robert Russell, MD, of Tufts' Jean Mayer USDA Human Nutrition Research Center on Aging, caution against relying on supplements as an "insurance policy" against an imperfect diet. It's better instead to eat a balanced and varied diet, from a wide variety of food groups.

To learn more: "What We Eat in America," Alanna Moshfegh, Joseph Goldman and Linda Cleveland, USDA Agricultural Research Service <www.ars.usda.gov/ Services/docs.htm?docid=9098>.

Lessons from New Guidelines and Pyramid

So how are we doing? The new federal dietary guidelines and high-tech food pyramid sparked a flurry of media attention in 2005. But since then it's been up to us to put the government's advice into practice, changing our diets and behavior.

You might conclude that we're not doing so hot. A report by the US Department of Health and Human Services (HHS), "Health, United States 2005," particularly sounds the alarm about the oldest vanguard of the Baby Boomers, those now ages 55 to 64: "Looking at their experience shows that risk factors like obesity and hypertension are going in the wrong direction," warns Amy Bernstein, director of the report and chief of the analytical studies branch at the National Center for Health Statistics. She notes that 40% of adults 55 to 64 are now obese, up from 31% just two years ago. While two-thirds of high-school students exercise regularly, the report found that only a third remain physically active as adults.

The report does have some good news: Life expectancy at birth has hit an all-time high, at 77.6 years; deaths from heart disease, stroke and cancer have declined 2% to 5%.

Of course, it's unrealistic to expect new dietary guidelines to change Americans' behavior so quickly, and many of the HHS report's statistics were actually gathered before the guidelines' unveiling. But the data does spotlight the challenge we face as increasingly overweight and sedentary citizens.

Eric Hentges, PhD, executive director of the US Agriculture Department's (USDA) Center for Nutrition Policy and Promotion, nonetheless believes we're off to a good start. "I'm very encouraged about the acceptance of the new guidelines and MyPyramid," he says, citing proprietary polling that found more than 70% of Americans approve of the government setting dietary standards. The same survey found a large majority had heard of the revised guidelines and had a generally positive reaction.

The real test is translating that favorable reception into action, Hentges adds. About a third of those surveyed said the new guidelines would make them change their habits, another third said they might change, and a third said they wouldn't alter their lifestyles. "That's about what we'd expect."

In its first nine months, the new MyPyramid Web site <www.mypyramid.gov> recorded 1.2 billion hits. More than a half-million people have signed up to use the site's interactive diet tracker, which lets users compare what they eat against the pyramid's plan. Educators have also jumped on board, with a 40% increase in tracker usage the first week of school.

Plus, Hentges says, "We've been very pleased with the way the pyramid has been incorporated in all the major scientific meetings."

He's also been pleasantly surprised by the food industry's embrace of the new recommendations. "They've really adopted a 'better for you' marketing mindset," Hentges says. "It's a growing phenomenon, incorporating the pyramid. The major food companies have billions of dollars in sales focused on this."

The most notable area where marketing has aligned with the government recommendations has been the boom in whole grains. In a significant departure from previous recommendations, the new guidelines call for half of all daily grain servings to come from whole-grain foods. Food manufacturers anticipated that change with a slew of new products and labels touting whole grains—nearly 100 new whole-grain products in 2004 alone—and customers seem to be buying: According to a report from the USDA's Economic Research Service, in the eight weeks after the guidelines' release, the average shopper bought about 13% more pounds of whole-grain products than for the same period the year before. Whole-grain bread purchases increased nearly 12%, whole-grain rice (such as brown rice) by almost 19%, and ready-to-eat cereals labeled as whole grains by 16%.

The "Power of Cheese" vs. the Power of Exercise

But US consumers still get mixed messages about nutrition from government and the food industry, says Alice H. Lichtenstein, DSc, Gershoff Professor at Tufts' Friedman School of Nutrition Science and Policy, who was on the panel that revised the dietary guidelines in 2000. Even as we're being told to increase whole grains and limit saturated fat, the American Dairy Association advertises "the power of cheese." Says Lichtenstein, "That's not a particularly helpful message if we're trying to tell people to reduce saturated fat. We have yet to see anything that says, 'Ahh, what a zucchini!'"

Those conflicting communications are among the reasons, she says, Americans have continued to battle obesity, heart disease and other problems since the federal dietary guidelines were first released in 1980. In the subsequent quarter-century, she points out, Americans have actually increased their intake of sugar, cheese, total fat and total calories. Some foods recommended in the guidelines—fish, fruits and vegetables—have, however, also seen modest increases in consumption. While whole milk consumption has dropped, that hasn't been completely counterbalanced by an increase in reduced-fat milk consumption, leaving Americans with a dairy deficit. Unfortunately, Lichtenstein notes, soda has filled the gap.

Perhaps most troubling, we've increasingly become couch potatoes. "As people get older, the percentage reporting no leisure-time physical activity has increased," Lichtenstein says.

The 2005 guidelines tackled that problem head-on, advising a minimum of 30 minutes' exercise daily (previously the basic recommendation) for general good health. To keep from gaining weight, however, the new standard is 60 minutes a day of moderate to vigorous exercise. And if you're looking to take off pounds, you'll need 90 minutes a day of physical activity.

Those facts about physical activity have been the toughest thing for most people to swallow about the new guidelines, Hentges concedes. "The reality of that strikes people kind of hard," he says. "People go, 'Holy smokes!' It's a reality check—that's what the science says. If you get up, go to work, are tired at the end of the day and just sit on the couch—if you don't go to the gym or do something else—then you're sedentary."

If you're not sure about your level of physical activity, Hentges suggests wearing a pedometer to count your steps for a few days. "Lots of us around here at the USDA have tried wearing pedometers. That pedometer will tell you if you're a sedentary person."

Unpuzzling Potassium, "Servings"

Other key recommendations of the new guidelines and pyramid may be easier for people to adopt, but challenges remain. The 2005 recommendations for the first time emphasized not only reducing sodium intake but also consuming potassium-rich foods, for instance. "Most people know that there's potassium in bananas, but not much else," says Lichtenstein. "The word 'potassium' is even a little scary, and if they see the chemical symbol 'K' for potassium, they don't make the connection."

The good news? If you eat enough fruits and vegetables, you likely don't have to worry about meeting the daily requirement for potassium intake.

Getting enough fruits and vegetables, though, can seem daunting based on the new recommendations, which call for nine daily servings. "What's a 'serving'? People need to keep in mind that a 'serving' size is modest," Lichtenstein says. "Frequently, the average serving these days is really two to three servings on the basis of the old pyramid."

For the first time in 2005, the guidelines talked as much in terms of "cups" as the often-confusing "servings." For fruits and vegetables, a serving is only a half-cup. So the call for nine daily servings translates into a recommendation of two cups of fruit and two and a half cups of vegetables a day, in a basic 2,000-calorie diet.

That doesn't all have to come from the fresh-produce section of your supermarket, Lichtenstein emphasizes. "Frozen vegetables are one of the best options for people," she says. "They're inexpensive, easy to store and can be used as needed." In fact, she adds, frozen vegetables often retain essential nutrients better than fresh, which can start to deteriorate on the grocer's shelf or in your refrigerator; frozen vegetables also avoid the salt that's often added in processing canned vegetables. Although frozen fruit, such as berries, lacks the texture of fresh produce, Lichtenstein says, it can be blended into smoothies or added to reduced-fat yogurt. And frozen fruit omits the extra sugar that canned-food processors often put in.

What's Next

Think you've figured out the 2005 federal dietary guidelines at last? That's good, because the whole process will crank up again sometime in 2008, Hentges says, for the next official update to be released in 2010. (By law, the Dietary Guidelines for Americans must be updated every five years.) The pyramid has been revised less frequently, only as needed; last year's simultaneous updating, as well as the close linking of the guidelines and MyPyramid, was unusual.

"The science behind the guidelines evolves at its own pace," Hentges adds. "We could probably go 10 years if everybody just stuck with the big scientific findings. But we need to revise every five years because there are a lot of other issues that come up, things like fad diets and other issues of society that are not yet necessarily ready for prime-time science. People need to have confidence in the consistency of the federal guidelines."

In the meantime, Lichtenstein hopes the public can get a clear message about nutrition and health. She advocates the creation of a "nutrition czar" position to unify nutrition policy. "We need to focus on the general public," she says. "This needs to permeate all aspects of society."

With a busy year of promoting the new guidelines and MyPyramid behind him, Hentges is also looking ahead. "The real question is: What happens in year two, year three?" he says. "We have to keep our eye on the long term, on how we help people make these healthy lifestyle changes."

To learn more: The complete dietary guidelines are available free online at <www.healthierus.gov/dietaryguidelines>. The free, interactive MyPyramid is at <www.mypyramid.gov>.

What's New?

Uncle Sam's information explosion about healthy food and lifestyle choices didn't stop with the release of the new dietary guidelines and MyPyramid in early 2005. Since then, the government has also spread the word with:

• *A Healthier You*, a new consumer-oriented book on healthy living, based on the 2005 guidelines. The book includes eating plans with nearly 100 recipes, ideas on using food labels, tips on physical activity, Web sites and worksheets, plus a foreword by First Lady Laura Bush. It's available for $15 in bookstores or directly from the Government Printing Office online at <bookstore.gpo.gov/collections/healthier_you.html> or by calling toll-free (866) 512-1800.

• MyPyramid for Kids and the MyPyramid Blast Off Game were launched online at <www.mypyramid.gov/kids>; the game got 260 million hits in its first two and a half months.

• A Spanish-language version of MyPyramid at <www.mypyramid.gov/sp-index.html> got 2 million hits in its first week and a half and accounted for 20% of traffic to the MyPyramid site.

Fruits & Veggies: New Program Says More Is Better

Forget "5-A-Day." Nutrition science "has just rocketed past" that familiar program designed to push produce consumption, says Dave Parker, director of marketing at Fruit Patch Sales and immediate past board chairman of the Produce for Better Health Foundation (PBH). The foundation, in partnership with the Centers for Disease Control (CDC), has been plastering the "5-A-Day" message on everything from blueberry baskets to school pencils since the early 1990s.

But the 2005 federal dietary guidelines call for as many as 13 half-cup servings of fruits and vegetables daily, and in fact largely drop that confusing "servings" terminology. So still talking about five daily servings—two and a half cups—of produce just didn't make sense, says Parker: "We knew we were in trouble. 5-A-Day wasn't viable anymore."

That's why in March 2007 the Produce for Better Health Foundation and the CDC will officially roll out a new program to encourage Americans to eat what's good for us: "Fruits & Veggies—More Matters." You'll start seeing the new slogan and logo on packages and promotions over the coming months, leading up to the formal launch.

The new message suggests that even if you aren't eating as much produce as the dietary guidelines advise—and can't seem to reach that target yet—more is still better. Whatever your current consumption, strive to fit more produce into your daily diet—an extra banana as a morning snack, another handful of vegetables in your stew.

"Our goal is to create an environment where consumers can change their behavior and include fruits and vegetables at every eating occasion," says Elizabeth Pivonka, president of the PBH.

Why More Matters for Health

While boosting produce consumption obviously benefits members of the industry-funded PBH, it also pays off for Americans' health. Says Pivonka, "Science indicates increased daily consumption of fruits and vegetables may help prevent many chronic diseases."

Research suggests that produce may help prevent some cancers, fight heart disease and diabetes and protect against macular degeneration in the eyes. Recent studies published in the *American Journal of Clinical Nutrition* have linked higher produce intake to reduced risk of cardiovascular disease and stroke and to better bone health. Eating plenty of fruits and vegetables also seems to help against obesity—and not only because you have less room in your diet for unhealthy snacks and high-fat foods: Another recent study in the *American Journal of Clinical Nutrition* showed that among 7,356 adults, those consuming 4.5 cups of produce or more daily were less likely to be obese, even if they also ate a diet high in fat.

Fruits and vegetables may even help your brain stay sharp. For example, Tufts nutrition researcher James Joseph, PhD, has found that blueberries can boost weakened neuron signals—resulting in improved short-term memory, navigational skills, balance, coordination and speed.

Phytonutrients in plant pigments, which give fruits and vegetables their color, also give the human body a healthful dose of antioxidants. The lycopene that makes tomatoes red may be effective against prostate cancer, for instance.

For optimum health benefits, it's important to eat a "rainbow" of fruits and vegetables, according to Joseph, co-author of the book *The Color Code: A Revolutionary Eating Plan for Optimum Health.* That book helped transform the "5-A-Day" campaign to "5-A-Day the Color Way."

Beyond French Fries

When the 5-A-Day campaign—originally a 1988 California-only promotion—first went nationwide, Americans' average produce consumption was only about 2.5 half-cup servings daily. Doubling that seemed like a worthy goal. Despite the omnipresence of the 5-A-Day message, however, a recent NPD Foodworld national survey found that only 20% of consumers actually meet even that modest target. And 96% of children ages 2-12 aren't getting enough fruits and vegetables.

When we do put produce on the plate, our choices leave much to be desired, nutritionally. According to the CDC, potatoes (often consumed as French fries), corn and peas account for 40% of the vegetables Americans eat. The 2005 dietary guidelines put a particular emphasis on increasing consumption of dark green leafy vegetables, such as spinach and kale, along with broccoli.

To try to get Americans' food preferences moving in the right direction, the new "Fruits & Veggies—More Matters" campaign was developed after a year of research and testing with more than 1,000 consumers. Even the phrasing "veggies" versus "vegetables" was tested; "veggies" scored better as "friendlier, fun and less formal."

The bottom line couldn't be simpler, though: Eat more fruits and "veggies." Says the PBH's Pivonka, "We wanted to be sure that the message was encouraging, and communicated that eating more is better for you, with an emphasis on making improvements to your diet even if you don't meet the specific recommendation."

To learn more: Produce for Better Health Foundation <www.pbhfoundation.org>.
My Pyramid <www.mypyramid.gov>.

Watermelon Nutrients Like It Warm

Want to get the most nutrition out of that juicy watermelon? Don't keep it in the fridge. Despite the picnic popularity of ice-cold watermelon, US Department of Agriculture (USDA) researchers report that watermelons stored at room temperature have substantially more nutrients than refrigerated or even freshly picked melons. Watermelons are rich in lycopene, an antioxidant that helps color their insides red; the USDA researchers found that melons continue to develop lycopene, as well as beta-carotene, after picking–but not if they're cold. Watermelons kept at 70 degrees Fahrenheit had as much as 40% more lycopene and 139% more beta-carotene, which the body converts to vitamin A, as fruit right off the vine. That nutrient development was slowed in refrigerated melons, which also decayed at least twice as fast.

Smarter–and Healthier–Supermarket Shopping Made Simple

With all the health claims on packaged goods these days and the countless news stories about "super foods," it would be easy to start thinking of your local supermarket as a sort of annex to your doctor's office. Just fill up your cart with "100% Whole Grain Goodness" and "Cholesterol-Fighting Power!" and you can skip that trip to the drugstore, right?

Well, not exactly. While you can find plenty of nutritious foods at your neighborhood supermarket, most grocery stores don't make it easy. Many packaged-goods health claims are confusing or misleading, and may paper over products that are also packed with sugar or sodium. And since supermarkets are designed to make you spend money, after all, your grocery cart's path of least resistance is more likely to lead to soda pop than to broccoli.

Marion Nestle, PhD, MPH, a professor of nutrition, food studies and public health at New York University, recently spent a year studying America's supermarkets, armed with a notebook and calculator, to research her new book, *What to Eat: An Aisle-by-Aisle Guide to Savvy Food Choices and Good Eating* (North Point Press, $30). As she's been interviewed to promote her book, Nestle regularly makes the point that supermarkets want customers to spend as much time as possible wandering their aisles. The more products you see, the more you are likely to buy.

But supermarkets don't necessarily give prominent placement to the healthiest foods, Nestle adds: "Products in the best locations—eye level, ends of aisles, cash registers—sell best. So companies pay the supermarkets to slot their products in prime real estate. These products are mostly junk because they are the most profitable and most heavily advertised."

Food companies spend $12 billion a year on direct media advertising, according to Nestle. Kellogg spends $32 million annually just on advertising its Cheez-Its snack crackers. For every dollar spent on ads, companies spend another two on trade shows, couponing and other promotions.

A typical 48,000-square-foot supermarket might contain 50,000 different items for sale. On average, a quarter of that store space is devoted to products that have added sugar, Nestle says.

In a *Washington Post* interview, Nestle recounted one of her supermarket research trips: "I was in an enormous one in Los Angeles. I couldn't help noticing that soft drinks were everywhere—a wall of them when you first walk in the store. Five aisles end with enormous soft-drink displays. Soft drinks next to the fish counter, near the garden furniture. You couldn't possibly go through the store without buying soft drinks."

Even if you're just popping in to buy a gallon of milk, Nestle says, you have to run a gauntlet of sweetened, salty and fatty treats to get to the dairy case—which savvy supermarkets strategically place all the way in the back.

Dried-fruit downsides

Q In a recent issue, you talk about the huge amounts of sugar in dried cranberries (such as Craisins). I had no idea. I particularly like, and eat on my cereal every morning, dried blueberries. I'm afraid to ask, but really would like to know if dried blueberries are the same? Also you said that the vitamin C was very low in dried cranberries–is that true of other dried fruit?

A While dried fruit is convenient, lasts long in your pantry and makes a tasty treat, it's no substitute for fresh fruit (or frozen fruit, if there's no added sugar) in your diet. Many dried fruits are sold sweetened, so you're getting extra sugar (or, more likely, high-fructose corn syrup). And the drying process does tend to deplete vitamin C—sometimes dramatically. One-third cup of fresh cranberries, for example, has 4.2 milligrams of vitamin C; even though it takes many more cranberries to make one-third cup of dried fruit—because so much water is removed—that serving size retains only 0.1 milligram of vitamin C. Plus you're getting 26 grams of sugar. Sorry, but the story's pretty much the same for dried blueberries: One popular brand has less than two percent of your daily vitamin C in a one-third-cup serving, with 24 grams of sugar. Check the list of ingredients; in this case, after blueberries the second ingredient listed is high-fructose corn syrup.

Dried fruit does retain some essential nutrients, however. Dried apricots, prunes, currants, cherries, figs and dates are good sources of potassium, as well as being high in fiber.

Patrol the Perimeter

So what's a health-conscious supermarket customer to do? In their book *Strong Women, Strong Hearts* (Putnam's, $25.95), Miriam E. Nelson, PhD, and Alice H. Lichtenstein, DSc, both on the faculty of Tufts' Friedman School, advocate "keeping the emphasis on the whole foods available on the perimeter of the supermarket (the produce and dairy aisles, for instance) rather than on the boxed, bagged, canned and other packaged goods lining all the center aisles. Those choices often contain too little fiber, too many refined carbohydrates that lack certain nutrients, and frequently too much in the way of sugar, saturated and trans fats and salt."

To peel or not to peel?

Q You reported on the importance of eating the peel of the Red Delicious apple. What about the peel of other fruits and vegetables, such as pears, peaches, tomatoes, grapes, blueberries, oranges and lemons, baked potato, kiwi, mango, papaya or carrots?

A In terms of the distribution of healthful polyphenolic phyto-chemicals such as flavonoids, yes, the skin, peel or outer layer of most plant foods is a particularly rich location for these compounds, according to Jeffrey Blumberg, PhD, chief of the Antioxidants Research Laboratory at Tufts' Jean Mayer USDA Human Nutrition Research Center on Aging. That's true in part because they serve as phytoalexins— defending the plant against fungus, insects, mold, ultraviolet light and other threats. The bran of grains and skin of tree nuts are also rich sources of these compounds. But Blumberg cautions, "Many of these compounds can also be quite astringent and/or bitter, thus the phytochemicals in the rind of lemons and oranges are normally not consumed (except as 'zest')." He also warns against any general rule to "always eat the skin," as some pesticide residue may be concentrated in the skin of fruits and vegetables.

You'll also generally get more dietary fiber if you eat the outer layer. A baked potato with the skin, for example, contains 4.6 grams of fiber; discarding the skin throws away half of that fiber. A medium apple with the skin has 3.3 grams of dietary fiber, while a peeled apple has just 1.7 grams of fiber. The benefits of 2.4 grams of fiber, however, probably don't justify chowing down on a quarter-cup of orange zest.

Demand Nutrient Density

Look instead for foods that are "nutrient dense." Eileen Kennedy, DSc, RD, dean of Tufts' Friedman School, explains, "They're the foods that are loaded with the nutrients we need to thrive. Think about choosing a potato instead of potato chips, or a banana instead of a soda. Opt for a plate with lots of vegetables, and skip the dinner roll. Ignore the cake and go for the fruit.

"If Americans choose foods based on nutrient density," Kennedy adds, "they will, essentially, be choosing foods based on quality." A food item that is nutrient-dense is generally a better choice than a less nutrient-dense item with the same number of calories.

As a rule, whole-grain breads and cereals are more nutrient-dense than their "white" counterparts. Many fruits and vegetables are nutrient-dense because, in addition to providing some basic carbohydrates, they are low in fat and packed with fiber, vitamins and minerals. Candy and sweetened beverages, in contrast, provide the carbohydrates (and maybe fats) without the other nutrients.

Read and Decode Nutrition Labels

Those "Nutrition Facts" food labels can be a grocery shopper's best friend, if you know how to read them. US law requires food labels on all processed foods; products with little nutritional value, such as coffee, don't have the labels, but do get freshness labels ("sell by" date). In a series of programs including "Supermarket Tour for Elders: No Cart Required!" at Tufts' Jean Mayer USDA Human Nutrition Research Center on Aging, speakers bureau coordinator Jean Bianchetto, RD, LDN, MS, goes through the Nutrition Facts label, line by line. The top section lists substances that Bianchetto says you should limit, such as fat, cholesterol and sodium. The bottom part lists minerals, such as calcium and iron, and vitamins that you should try to include in your diet. The daily value percentages on the label are based on a daily intake of 2,000 calories. Bianchetto notes that 5% of the daily value is considered low, while 20% or more is considered high.

Making a List

To make your own grocery list of foods certified as heart-healthy by the American Heart Association, go online to <checkmark.heart.org>. You can build your list searching by manufacturer or food category. A handy "My Items" feature lets you type in household items like soap or cat litter that you also need to buy. Then simply select "Print List" and head for the store. (Be aware, though, Marion Nestle points out, that the heart association seal signifies only that a product is low in fat and cholesterol; it could still contain lots of added sugar.)

Center-Aisle Survival Tips

If you do stray into the packaged-goods aisles in the center of the supermarket, Nestle has a litany of "rules" that can help:
- Don't buy anything with more than five ingredients.
- If you can't pronounce the ingredients on the package label, don't buy it.
- Don't buy anything with a cartoon on it—it's being advertised directly to your kids or grandkids.

- If you don't want your kids eating junk food, don't have it in your house.
- Don't buy artificial anything—it's just disguising bad taste.

She also cautions against buying foods that seem like health foods—but really aren't. Just because candy comes covered with yogurt, for example, doesn't make it good for you. Also skip the "power bars" and "energy drinks" that purport to help athletes refuel; they're loaded with sweeteners and extra calories. "And don't buy anything with claims for health benefits. These are out of context and you need to search for the qualifying statements in tiny print."

Of course, it is possible to buy foods that are good for you in those temptation-packed center aisles. That's where you'll usually find whole-grain products, for example, as well as frozen and canned fruits and vegetables. But be careful and scrutinize labels to make sure that grains and healthy produce are all that you're buying.

Consider the aisle where many supermarkets sell not only rice and sometimes specialty grains but also packaged rice dishes. You probably already know that brown rice—a whole grain—is better for you than white rice. But what about those tasty-looking boxes of "rice pilaf"? Though they might sound like a good source of grain, a cup contains a mere 1 gram of fiber—along with 9 grams of total fat, 2 grams of saturated fat and a whopping 1,180 milligrams of sodium, almost half your daily total. Plus you're piling more than 300 calories onto your plate.

Similar cautions apply over in the cereal aisle, where you can buy a box of oatmeal that's all whole grains and nothing but. You might be tempted, though, by the Peanut Butter Toast Crunch cereal—after all, the box says in huge letters, as big as the words "Toast Crunch," "Whole Grain." Sure enough, the first ingredient listed is whole grain wheat. But keep reading, remembering that ingredients are listed in order by weight: Sugar comes next, followed by "creamy peanut butter" made with, yes, sugar, then rice flour and then fructose (another kind of sugar), and a bit farther down is dextrose (yet another kind of sugar). A serving has 10 grams of sugars in all. What about Maple Pecan Crunch cereal, "inspired by the taste of home-baked maple pecan muffins" and an "excellent source of Whole Grain"? It lists oats and then brown sugar, with plain sugar sixth on the ingredients list. Despite the whole-grain claims and homey-goodness appeal, a bowl contains 13 grams of sugars and 6 of fat.

Nothing says you can't indulge in an occasional muffin—or a cereal that tastes like a muffin. Just don't be fooled into thinking it's health food.

Pick Produce with Care

Frozen and canned fruits and vegetables found in supermarket center aisles can be affordable, convenient alternatives to fresh produce, but here too you need to give products a checkup before they go into your cart. Frozen produce is less likely to have added salt or sugar, and fruits and vegetables generally lose fewer nutrients in freezing than canning. Stick to canned goods that are as close to the whole, unprocessed original as possible, without added salt or sugar. The more food preparation and flavoring that a packager does for you, the more likely you're buying ingredients you may not want, at least in such quantities: A serving of canned barbecue baked beans, for instance, has 510 milligrams of sodium and 13 grams of sugars—in fact, sugar is the third ingredient listed, after water and beans.

Super Ideas for the Supermarket

Get a jump start on groceries with this list of recommended pantry staples and other basics of healthy food shopping from the National Heart, Lung and Blood Institute:

Fat-free or low-fat milk, yogurt, cheese and cottage cheese

Eggs/egg substitutes

Breads, bagels, pita bread, English muffins (whole grain)

Low-fat flour tortillas

Cereal (whole-grain)

Rice (such as brown rice, or other whole grains)

Pasta (look for whole-grain pasta)

White meat chicken or turkey (remove skin)

Fish and shellfish (fresh or frozen, not battered)

Beef: round, sirloin, chuck arm, loin and extra-lean ground beef

Pork: leg, shoulder, tenderloin

Dry beans and peas

Fresh, frozen, canned fruits in light syrup or juice

Fresh, frozen or no-salt-added canned vegetables

Low-fat or nonfat salad dressings

Herbs and spices

Now take another look at that can of beans: The serving size is a half-cup. When you have baked beans, how much do you really put on your plate? A typical soup ladle (not heaping) serves about a half-cup. If you take two or three ladles of beans, you need to adjust your thinking accordingly when studying labels at the store.

Even vegetarian meals from those center aisles can be nutritionally iffy. A serving of frozen fettucini alfredo, for example, though meatless, nonetheless has 450 calories, 12 grams of saturated fat and 910 milligrams of sodium—more than a three-ounce lean hamburger including the bun.

So stick to the edges of the supermarket when possible, and always look at labels. Before you check out, remember to give your grocery cart a check-up.

Everybody's Going Organic– Should You?

The answer: It depends. Here's how to know when to consider buying organic—and when to save your money.

IF YOU'VE BEEN down the aisles of your local grocery store recently, chances are you've noticed the addition or expansion of "organic" items. Eyeing the success of specialty retailers like Whole Foods and Wild Oats Market, which focus on the "natural" and organic grocery niche, conventional retailers are angling to cash in on the growing organic trend. Even mega-retailer Wal-Mart recently hopped on the organic bandwagon, bringing in new lines of products and devoting increased shelf space to organic items. Industry analysts say growth in the organic food and product segment has been "explosive"—increasing up to 20% annually nationwide in recent years. Organic products now total more than $10 billion in annual consumer sales, according to the Organic Trade Association.

After it was determined that a patchwork quilt of state regulations was not protecting the public's interests, in 2003 the US Department of Agriculture (USDA) finalized national standards for foods and products claiming to be "organic." Items labeled "certified organic" must pass a clearly defined certification process, with federal agents visiting and inspecting the farms, feedlots, manufacturing plants and even retailers that wish to boast the organic label. In a nutshell, certified organic foods cannot be genetically modified or irradiated; produce cannot be farmed with most synthetic pesticides or fertilizers; and organic dairy, poultry, meat and eggs are produced without growth hormones and antibiotics.

Although organic foods are sometimes equivalent in price to conventionally produced items, they typically cost from 25% more to even *double* the price of regular products. Why are so many of us "going organic," despite the price tag? And are organic foods really worth it in terms of contributing to better health and nutrition?

Why go organic?

Concerns about pesticides lead the list of reasons consumers are increasingly looking to organic alternatives. Currently, more than 400 chemicals can be used in conventional farming to kill weeds, insects and other pests that attack crops. For example, some (non-organic) apples are sprayed up to 16 times with 36 different pesticides.

Fruits and Veggies Rated a Nutritional Bargain

LOOKING FOR THE BEST nutritional bang for your buck? Buy fruits and vegetables, says a team of French and US researchers who analyzed 637 foods using a nutrient-to-price ratio. Produce topped their list for providing "essential nutrients at a reasonable price." Among the best-scoring fruits and vegetables in nutrient density per dollar were oranges, bananas, carrots, cabbage, tomatoes, zucchini, celery, onions, canned mixed vegetables and fruit juices. Not far behind were lean meats and dairy products. Below-average scores went to grains, meats in general and composite dishes such as pizza or spaghetti and meatballs. The worst values in nutrients for the money? Desserts and other sweets.

To learn more: *Journal of the American Dietetic Association*, Dec. 2005. Free abstract at <www.adajournal.org/ article/ PIIS000282 230501552X/abstract>.

A number of recent studies have shown possible links between pesticides and serious disease. The most dangerous chemicals used in farming, such as the pesticides known as organophosphates, have been linked with higher incidences of certain types of cancer, male infertility and Parkinson's disease. Researchers at the National Cancer Institute, the National Institute of Environmental Health Sciences and the Environmental Protection Agency found in a study that farmers and nursery workers who use certain pesticides have a higher-than-average risk of prostate cancer. Women with breast cancer are five to nine times more likely to have pesticide residues in their blood than those who do not.

Buying organic may make sense especially for those concerned about the health effects of pesticides on their children and grandchildren, according to research at the University of Washington. Children eating non-organic foods were switched to an organic diet for five days, and pesticide levels were measured in their urine before and after the change. The study found that some pesticides disappeared from the children's urine after going organic.

"We don't say that moving to more organic food will necessarily change your risk," researcher Richard Fenske, PhD, told the *Seattle Post-Intelligencer*. "But it will change your children's pesticide exposure."

Fenske, a professor with the UW's School of Public Health and one of the researchers on the study, previously published results showing that children consuming produce and juice grown using conventional farming practices had urine levels of some pesticide types that were five to seven times higher than for children with a largely organic diet. The study stopped short of defining what long-term health effects, if any, may be triggered by consuming low levels of pesticides. But other research has shown that eating organic does reduce the amount of toxic chemicals ingested, enables the consumer to totally avoid genetically modified organisms (GMOs), and reduces the intake of food additives, such as colorings and preservatives.

Additionally, some research has shown that foods grown organically actually have higher levels of beneficial vitamins, minerals, essential fatty acids and antioxidants, nutrients thought to slow the aging process. And in some studies, eating organic seems to lower the incidence of diseases, such as cancer and coronary heart disease, and even reduce the occurrence of allergies.

Worth paying extra?

But none of this means organic food is always your best or smartest buy. According to Consumers Union and other independent researchers, sometimes it may be worth the extra cost to buy organic food products to reduce your exposure to pesticides and other additives. Other times, it might be beneficial but not essential to go organic. And there are times, the independent researchers concur, that it's simply a waste of your money.

Best bets to buy organic:

Apples, bell peppers, celery, cherries, imported grapes, nectarines, peaches, pears, potatoes, red raspberries, spinach, strawberries—Some fruits and vegetables carry much higher levels of pesticide residue than others, even after careful washing. This was verified by testing in USDA laboratories. Researchers at the Environmental Working Group (EWG), a public watchdog group that's advocated for organic farming, developed this list they call the "dirty dozen"—fruits and vegetables they say you should always buy organic if possible because of pesticide residue in their conventionally grown counterparts.

Beef, poultry, eggs and dairy—Consumers Union says it's worth the extra money to buy organic beef because you greatly reduce the risk of exposure to the agent that causes mad-cow disease. The organization also recommends buying organic poultry, eggs and dairy products, saying you'll avoid ingesting supplemental hormones and antibiotics, which have been linked to increased antibacterial resistance in humans.

Baby food—Children's developing bodies are especially vulnerable to toxins. Baby food is often made up of condensed fruits or vegetables, potentially concentrating pesticide residues.

Only marginal benefits buying organic:

Asparagus, avocados, bananas, broccoli, cauliflower, sweet corn, kiwi, mangos, onions, papaya, pineapples, sweet peas—Multiple pesticide residues are rarely found on conventionally grown versions of these fruits and vegetables, according to research by the EWG. You can save money by buying the conventional versions of these produce items with no substantial risk of pesticide exposure.

Breads, oils, snack foods, pasta, cereals and other packaged foods, such as canned or dried fruit and vegetables—Although the organic versions of these processed products may have lower levels of contaminants, they offer limited added health value. That's especially true of packaged foods that aren't that good for you in the first place: A potato chip is still a potato chip, organic or not. Also, processed products by their very nature include a multitude of ingredients: Reading the label on a "Made with organic ingredients" product, you'll probably find that while the flour is organic, other ingredients aren't.

Don't bother buying organic:

Seafood—The USDA has not yet developed organic certification standards for seafood. Whether caught in the wild or farmed, fish can be labeled "organic," despite the presence of contaminants such as mercury and PCBs, a serious concern with some fish consumption. Additionally, producers are allowed to make their own organic claims as long as they don't use "USDA" or "certified organic" logos.

Cosmetics—Unless a personal-care product consists primarily of organic agricultural ingredients, such as aloe vera gel, independent researchers say it's pointless to buy organic in this category. Most cosmetics contain a mix of ingredients, and USDA regulations allow shampoos and body lotions to carry an "organic" label even when water is the primary ingredient. Making informed decisions and buying organic products that are ingested, the researchers say, is a much higher health priority, so don't take a bath on pricey "organic" shampoo.

To learn more: *Environmental Health Perspectives*, March 2003; abstract at <www.ehponline.org/docs/ 2003/5754/abstract.html>. Organic Trade Association <www.ota.com>. Environmental Working Group <www.ewg.org> and <www.foodnews.org>. Consumers Union <www.consumersunion.org>.

Making the Most of Nutrition Facts Labels

New studies say many Americans are stumped by nutrition labels. How about you?

A new survey reports that more than half of us check nutritional labeling on product packaging before we buy, and two out of five adults say they have changed their eating habits to more closely follow the US Department of Agriculture's (USDA) My Pyramid nutrition recommendations. That's the good news.

But the Harris Interactive/*Wall Street Journal* survey also revealed that a surprising percentage of Americans—even well-educated people with good reading and math skills—don't know how to read and interpret the label data correctly.

The online survey involved almost 3,000 American adults, 95% of whom said they have at some point used products' nutritional labeling when making food decisions. The three most frequently cited reasons for consulting food labels were to follow a balanced, nutritious diet (39%), management of a medical condition such as diabetes or high cholesterol (23%) and weight loss (19%). Respondents listed their top three concerns as fat, calorie and sugar content.

But despite the fact that we're checking labels, a recent study indicates

---

Counting on Iron

Although the percentages on a Nutrition Facts label reflect a Daily Value of 18 milligrams of iron, for example, your actual daily need varies with age and gender. Here's what the Institute of Medicine most recently set in 2001 as Dietary Reference Intakes for iron per day:

Infants, 7-12 months–11 mg	Males, 19 and up–8 mg
Children, 1-3 years–7 mg	Females, 9-13–8 mg
Children, 4-8–10 mg	Females, 14-18–15 mg
Males, 9-13–8 mg	Females, 19-50–18 mg
Males, 14-18–11 mg	Females, 51 and up–8 mg

Pregnant women should get 27 milligrams daily and lactating women should get 9 milligrams (10 milligrams if age 14-18).

many Americans struggle with interpreting and applying that data on the side of the box. Researchers from Vanderbilt University Medical Center questioned 200 participants from a wide socioeconomic range, asking them to interpret food labels for nutrient content by the amount of food consumed. Another segment of the study asked participants to identify which foods had more or less of a certain nutrient.

Going into the study, most participants (89%) felt confident they understood nutritional labels and could use them to make healthy choices. But the study's results, published in the *American Journal of Preventive Medicine*, showed otherwise. The study uncovered a significant gap in the general public's understanding of nutrition-label information. And while poor label comprehension did correlate with lower literacy and mathematic skills, even better-educated participants sometimes stumbled.

Only 37% of participants could correctly calculate the total grams of carbohydrates in a 20-ounce bottle of soda that contained 2-1/2 servings. And when given the nutrition data on a whole bagel, only 60% could figure how many grams of carbohydrates they would consume if they ate only half a bagel.

Many participants were confused by the complexity of the nutrition label, the researchers found, and were unable to find the facts they needed to answer researchers' questions. Some subjects confused the nutritional values given for the product they were eating with the recommended values for the whole day, or mistakenly incorporated the percentage of the product's values as part of a 2,000-calorie recommended daily allowance (RDA).

One size doesn't fit all

To assist the nutrition label-reading public, the US Food and Drug Administration (FDA) is considering a number of modifications, including changes to the way calories, trans fats and portion sizes—three key factors in healthy eating—are listed on product packaging. An FDA food-labeling seminar held earlier this year pondered possible changes in how calorie content and portion sizes are reported.

But don't expect to see those changes anytime soon, says Jeanne P. Goldberg, PhD, a registered dietician and director of Tufts' Graduate Program in Nutrition Communication. A number of factors—the complexity of the issue, the amount of research that will need to be done and the number of health organizations and food-industry representatives who will want to weigh in on the topic—mean that it could be a while before we see different labels in supermarkets.

Goldberg was a member of a US/Canadian committee, convened in 2004 by the US Institute of Medicine, charged with making recommendations for revamping the Daily Values, a prime component of nutrition labels' information.

It's true, Goldberg says, that the current nutrition label format, issued in 1992, is based on standards established in 1968. It's not that the standards are necessarily outdated, but rather how they were determined. These were based on "highest estimated needs" from a much larger set of standards, the Recommended Dietary Allowances, which take into account the effect of such factors as age and sex in estimating recommendations.

There are big differences, in needs for some nutrients related to age and gender. Iron is a good example. The current nutrition standard for iron—18 milligrams—is based on the 1968 determination of the needs of women

---

The Devil Made Us Ignore that Nutrition Label!

ONE PROBLEM WITH using nutrition information to wage war on obesity turns out to have less to do with the labels themselves than with compliance. So says a new study by market-research firm AC Nielsen that found, frankly, Americans don't always do what we know we should, nutrition-wise.

While 82% of American adults acknowledged their individual responsibility in weight gain, consumers nevertheless tended to eat the "wrong" things for weight loss and maintenance. And although 65% of respondents agreed that reducing junk-food consumption would help them with weight control, and 61% thought it sage advice to drink water rather than sugary soft drinks, few consumers in the study said they actually followed this advice.

Asked why they went ahead and bought products they knew—by reading those Nutrition Facts labels—would pack on the pounds, many respondents faulted the "modern convenience culture," saying lifestyle changes associated with weight control just seemed too inconvenient to follow.

---

in their childbearing years. Depending on who you actually *are*—a full-grown male or senior woman, for example—18 milligrams of iron may supply anywhere from 120-257% of your actual daily need.

Looking beyond labels

How to fit all that on the panel of a cereal box or frozen lasagna? That's not really the point, Goldberg says. Consumers needn't wait for the ultimate nutritional label to start making healthier nutritional decisions, she maintains. "I feel we actually know more about how to eat right than we give ourselves credit for," Goldberg says. Instead of getting tripped up on percentages and RDAs, consumers should strive to build healthy eating habits by returning to "the basics," she explains. That means eating mostly basic foods and consuming fewer prepared foods—no math required.

You can leave your calculator at home if you "shop the perimeter" of the grocery store, Goldberg says. That's where the least-processed foods are shelved: produce, lean meat and poultry, seafood, dairy products. Moving into the inner aisles, yes, you can find good choices among some convenience foods, she says. In fact, convenience is crucial to many people as they try to choose healthier options. You should check the label to avoid high amounts of fat, calories and sodium, while seeking out packaged goods with higher fiber content.

Math may come in, of course, where healthy choices collide with high grocery prices. For example, fresh produce out of season can get frightfully expensive. Rather than cut back on vegetables, though, Goldberg advises consumers to buy frozen or canned when needed.

"There's nothing wrong with them. They are a perfectly good source of nutrition," she says, adding that consumers would do well to choose the plain frozen bagged broccoli over the package with high-fat cheddar cheese sauce.

Getting a handle on portion control is major component of learning to eat more healthfully, Goldberg notes. But that's a subject where consumers might need to pay closer attention.

"How many people know what two ounces of pasta looks like?" she asks. "The label tells you that two ounces is a portion. Is that a side dish? Is that if pasta is the main dish? I actually weigh my pasta before I cook it. It's the only way I can be sure to get a handle on it, and that's where consumers can make a big and positive change in their eating habits and the overall health of their diets."

To learn more: *American Journal of Preventive Medicine*, November 2006;
online at <www.ajpm-online.net/webfiles/images/journals/amepre/AMEPRE1755.pdf>.
USDA Food and Nutrition Information Center
<fnic.nal.usda.gov/nal_display/ index.php?info_center=4&tax_level=1&tax_subject=273>.
Institute of Medicine Dietary Reference Intakes <www.iom.edu/?id=37067>.

Decoding Nutrition Labels

Serving Size: This is the place to start when looking at the Nutrition Facts label. It tells you a normal portion and how many servings are in the package. Compare this portion size to how much you actually consume.

Calories provide a measure of how much energy you get from a serving of this food. Many Americans consume more calories than they need without meeting recommended intakes for a number of nutrients. The calorie section of the label can help you manage your weight. As a general guide, 40 calories per serving is low, 100 calories is moderate, and 400 or more is high.

The **nutrients** listed first are the ones Americans generally eat in adequate amounts— or, more often, to excess. Eating too much saturated fat, trans fat, cholesterol or sodium may increase your risk of certain chronic diseases, such as heart disease, some cancers or high blood pressure.

Note the **asterisk** after the heading "% Daily Value." It refers to the footnote in the lower part of the label, which tells you the percentages are based on a 2,000 calorie-a-day diet.

Most Americans don't get enough **dietary fiber, vitamin A, vitamin C, calcium and iron.** Eating enough of these nutrients can improve your health and help reduce the risk of some diseases and conditions.

The **Percent Daily Value** are based on the recommendations for key nutrients as calculated for a 2,000-calorie daily diet. Many people consume more calories in a day, and most don't even know how many calories they consume. But you can still use the percentages as a frame of reference, whether you consume more or fewer than 2,000 calories. (Source: US Food and Drug Administration)

Nutrition Facts

Serving Size 1 cup (228g)
Servings Per Container 2

Amount Per Serving

Calories 250   Calories from Fat 110

	% Daily Value*
Total Fat 12g	18%
Saturated Fat 3g	15%
Trans Fat 3g	
Cholesterol 30mg	10%
Sodium 470mg	20%
Total Carbohydrate 31g	10%
Dietary Fiber 0g	0%
Sugars 5g	
Protein 5g	

Vitamin A	4%
Vitamin C	2%
Calcium	20%
Iron	4%

* Percent Daily Values are based on a 2,000 calorie diet. Your Daily Values may be higher or lower depending on your calorie needs.

		Calories:	2,000	2,500
Total Fat	Less than		65g	80g
Sat Fat	Less than		20g	25g
Cholesterol	Less than		300mg	300mg
Sodium	Less than		2,400mg	2,400mg
Total Carbohydrate			300g	375g
Dietary Fiber			25g	30g

How Safe Are
Your Salad Greens?

Nutrition experts have been urging us to eat more leafy green vegetables for our health, but recent outbreaks of contaminated spinach and lettuce suddenly make that salad bowl seem scary instead of healthy. First, some 200 Americans in 26 states got sick and three died from E. coli bacteria in packaged spinach. Then, days later, lettuce packages were recalled in seven states after the grower found E. coli in its irrigation water. Frightened consumers were left wondering: How safe are supermarket greens? And what, if anything, can ordinary people do to combat salad contamination?

Most experts agree this largely unregulated industry has a ways to go before consumers can feel as confident about greens as, say, pasteurized milk. "The industry has to reinvent itself and get this fixed," says Mike Doyle, PhD, director of the University of Georgia Center for Food Safety.

On the other hand, the remote risk of contamination is no reason to panic or stop eating greens. Since 1995, the US Food and Drug Administration (FDA) says lettuce or spinach has been involved in 20 E. coli outbreaks. That's 20 too many, but a tiny portion of the $4.4 billion annual US lettuce and spinach industry.

Doyle, however, believes it is significant that the last nine outbreaks were associated with packaged greens, now 80% of the market. That's ironic, since consumers opt for packaged greens not only for convenience but for safety. But Doyle, who no longer buys packaged greens himself, says the process invites contamination: Lettuce gets cut and cored out in the field "with a long knife that's not disinfected in-between. That creates a wound that lets bacteria in, where they're next to impossible to remove." The outer layers, where microbes most likely lurk, are also discarded, exposing the edible leaves to contamination. Finally, in the packaging plant, contaminated greens can get mixed with clean ones.

"It's safer to buy whole heads of lettuce, remove the outer three layers yourself, then wash your hands," Doyle advises. "Then you can wash the inner layers and eat those. At least then you have control."

"Triple washing" in chlorinated water is supposed to kill bacteria in packaged greens. But it's not 100% effective even if done properly, which inspection records indicate isn't always the case.

Washing greens at home removes only 60-90% of microbes, according to Scientific Certification Systems, which audits produce-industry practices. As for so-called "vegetable washes," Richard Linton, director of Purdue University's Center for Food Safety Engineering, says supermarket products "are minimally effective. Most work about as well as a tap-water rinse."

The only sure way to eliminate bacteria, he says, is by cooking—not an option with lettuce, though a possibility for spinach.

Other greens—restaurants tried arugula after the spinach scare—aren't any less likely to be contaminated. "Most leafy vegetables that are in close association with the ground would have a similar risk," Linton adds. "I think we recognize the issues associated with lettuce and spinach mainly because of the mass distribution of these leafy greens. Growing practices for most leafy greens are very similar."

Nor is switching to organic greens a solution, according to Doyle. He cites a University of Minnesota study that found organic produce more likely to have indicators of E. coli contamination than conventional vegetables.

Nonetheless, both food-safety experts continue to eat salads. And Linton says he still buys packaged greens despite the recent scares, noting that the packaging protects greens from contamination during food distribution.

To learn more: FDA Center for Food Safety and Applied Nutrition <www.cfsan.fda.gov>.

You Are What You Drink: New Guidelines Give Beverage Advice

JUST BECAUSE that "sports drink" features athletes in its ads doesn't mean it's your healthiest choice to quench your thirst. In fact, a new proposed guidance system for beverage consumption ranks sports drinks near the bottom.

Americans now consume 21% of their daily calories from all beverages, up from 13-15% in the 1970s. While watching their plates, dieters often overlook the calories and fat in their glasses, cups and bottles.

"Many people either forget or don't realize how many extra calories they consume in what they drink, yet beverages are a major contributor to the alarming increase in obesity," says Barry Popkin, PhD, director of the University of North Carolina's Interdisciplinary Obesity Center, who led the development of the guidelines. "The Healthy Beverage Guidelines will show Americans the impact that liquid calories have on their overall diets, and help them make responsible beverage choices."

The experts' recommendations on the health and nutritional benefits and risks of various beverage categories were published in the *American Journal of Clinical Nutrition*. Much like the government's food pyramid, which suggests a balanced way of choosing different types of food for more healthful nutrition, the Healthy Beverage Guidelines provide a ranking system. Rankings range from plain water at Level One to Level Six—beverages that should be consumed in limited quantities. The guidelines are designed to help consumers choose a more balanced and healthful palette of beverages, based on sugar content, fat and caffeine, and caloric count.

The panel stressed that a healthy diet does not rely on fluids to provide energy or nutrient needs, and that water—necessary for metabolism and normal physiological function—is the only fluid truly needed by the body. For variety and individual preferences, however, healthful diets may include other beverages. Many Americans also need other beverages, such as 1% or nonfat milk, for essential nutrients.

The guidelines are hardly the only red flag that's been recently raised about what Americans are quaffing. A study published in *Pediatrics* found that teenage boys whose sugary soft-drinks were replaced with non-caloric drinks lost weight. The researchers noted that liquid calories can be "invisible" and don't alleviate hunger as effectively as solid food.

Other scientists, at the University of Florida, recently warned that so-called "energy drinks" contain caffeine at levels above the FDA limit for sodas (65 milligrams per 12 ounces)—a fact not disclosed on most labels. The caffeine in energy drinks tested ranged from 33 milligrams to an eye-popping 141 milligrams in a 16-ounce SoBe No Fear. Coffee drinks also packed more than the recommended punch, notably Starbucks' Doubleshot, with 105 milligrams of caffeine.

Is all this talk about beverages making you thirsty? We suggest you reach for a glass of good old *un*bottled water.

To learn more: *American Journal of Clinical Nutrition,* March 2006. Details of the full study online at <www.beverageguidancepanel.org>. *Pediatrics,* March 2006. *Journal of Analytical Toxicity,* 2006: 30.

Healthy Beverage Guidelines

LEVEL 1: WATER

The Beverage Guidance panel notes that all beverage needs for adults can be met with water.

Recommendation: 20-50 ounces per day.

LEVEL 2: UNSWEETENED TEA AND COFFEE

Tea provides a variety of flavonoids and antioxidants as well as a few micronutrients, and may have other health benefits. Current research suggests that moderate caffeine intake (up to 400 milligrams/day) is not associated with increased risk of heart disease, hypertension, osteoporosis or high cholesterol.

Recommendation: 0-40 ounces of unsweetened tea and 0-32 ounces of unsweetened coffee per day. Caffeine is the limiting factor, with twice as much in coffee as in tea.

LEVEL 3: LOW FAT (1.5% OR 1%) AND SKIM (NONFAT) MILK AND SOY BEVERAGES

Milk is an important source of calcium and the key dietary source of vitamin D. Fortified soymilk is a good alternative for individuals who prefer not to consume cow's milk.

Recommendation: 0-16 ounces a day.

LEVEL 4: NON-CALORICALLY SWEETENED BEVERAGES

Diet sodas and other sugar-free drinks are preferable to sugar-sweetened beverages because they provide no calories. FDA-approved non-caloric sweeteners are considered safe. **Recommendation:** 0-32 ounces per day.

LEVEL 5: CALORIC BEVERAGES WITH SOME NUTRIENTS

Fruit juices (100% juice) provide most of the nutrients of their natural source, but lack fiber and other beneficial non-nutrient compounds present in the whole fruit.

Recommendation: 0-8 ounces per day

Vegetable juices (e.g., tomato and multi-vegetable juices) are a healthy alternative; the trade-off is sugar for sodium, as many of these drinks are moderately high in sodium. **Recommendation:** 0-8 ounces per day

Whole (full fat) milk contains calcium and protein, but adverse health effects of saturated fats have been well documented, especially risk of cardiovascular disease. **Recommendation:** No whole milk.

Sports drinks do provide small amounts of sodium, chloride and potassium–replacing electrolytes lost during endurance activities–but that benefit is offset by the caloric content. **Recommendation:** Consume sparingly except for endurance athletes, 0-16 ounces per day.

Alcoholic beverages consumed in moderation have been shown to have some health benefits for adults, including reduced risk of cardiovascular disease, type 2 diabetes and gallstones. On the downside, even moderate intake of alcoholic beverages is linked with increased risk of birth defects and breast cancer. Pregnant women should not drink alcoholic beverages. Recommendation: 0-1 drink per day for women and 0-2 drinks per day for men (one drink is 12 ounces beer, 5 ounces wine, or 1.5 ounces distilled spirits).

LEVEL 6: CALORICALLY SWEETENED BEVERAGES WITHOUT NUTRIENTS

The least-recommended beverages by the panel are calorically sweetened beverages with little to no nutritional value. These include carbonated and non-carbonated beverages, usually sweetened with high-fructose corn syrup or sucrose. **Recommendation:** No more than one 8-ounce serving per day.

Can coffee count?

Q Many people talk about the dehydrating effects of caffeine. Just how much caffeine is dehydrating and how much is the water in it hydrating? How much do coffee and tea count toward getting enough water per day?

A A 2000 study at the University of Nebraska's Center for Human Nutrition put the supposed dehydrating powers of caffeine to the test on 18 adult males, ages 24 to 39. The results, published in the *Journal of the American College of Nutrition*, found no significant difference in the hydration effect of various combinations of beverages, including coffee and cola. The study's authors concluded, "Advising people to disregard caffeinated beverages as part of the daily fluid intake is not substantiated by the results of this study."

As we reported in the April 2004 *Healthletter*, this conclusion was confirmed as part of new water-consumption guidelines issued by an Institute of Medicine panel of distinguished US and Canadian scientists, convened by the National Academy of Sciences. That panel noted, "As early as 1928, it was reported that caffeine-containing beverages did not significantly increase 24-hour urine output," and found that any diuretic effects of caffeine are transient in nature. Those guidelines say that coffee, tea, colas and (in moderation) alcoholic beverages (subject of another dehydration myth) can contribute to total water intake. That's particularly true of habitual consumers of caffeinated beverages such as coffee, because your body adapts: The more regularly you drink it, the more the body is able to hold onto the water it provides

By the way, you can also stop counting glasses of water. The panel debunked the "eight glasses a day" goal and said that for most people, "fluid intake, driven by thirst… allows maintenance of hydration status and total body water at normal levels." In fact, a 2002 Dartmouth review of more than 30 years of nutrition studies found that the average daily water intake "of thousands of presumably healthy humans" was closer to four glasses.

Watching Your Waistline

Keep Your Weight Normal to Live Longer

The debate about weight and mortality has heated up again, with two hefty new studies providing scientific evidence for what most people have long suspected: It's better not to be too fat *or* too thin. The studies, both published in the *New England Journal of Medicine*, took particularly careful account of smoking and chronic illness, which can complicate the relationship between weight and early death. According to the findings, even a little extra weight increases your risk of death.

The studies run counter to controversial research earlier by the federal Centers for Disease Prevention and Control (CDC) and National Cancer Institute that seemed to link being slightly overweight with a reduced risk of death. CDC chief Julie Gerberding, MD, subsequently backed away from those findings, conceding that the results may have been skewed by including people with chronic diseases, who tend to weigh less but die early.

Almost simultaneous with the release of the two new studies linking abnormal weight and mortality risk, however, another pair of studies challenged the reliability of Body Mass Index (BMI) as a tool for predicting cardiovascular risk and for forecasting mortality in people over age 75. (See next section.) Both new studies connecting weight and mortality used BMI to measure over- and underweight and obesity. But even the researchers questioning BMI agreed that their findings don't mean it's OK to be fat; rather, the issue is how best to measure excess weight.

Weighing the evidence

In one of the *New England Journal of Medicine* studies, scientists followed 527,265 men and women, ages 50 to 71 when the study began, who were members of the AARP (formerly the American Association of Retired Persons) organization. The participants in the National Institutes of Health-AARP cohort filled out questionnaires in 1995 and 1996. Through 2005, 61,317 subjects had died. "Initial analyses showed an increased risk of death for the highest and lowest categories of BMI among both men and women, in all racial and ethnic groups, and at all ages," wrote senior author Michael F. Leitzman, MD, of the National Cancer Institute (NCI). Compared to participants with a BMI at the upper end of the "normal" range, 23.5 to 24.9, those who were underweight—BMI below 18.5—had a 50% greater risk of death.

When the researchers narrowed their focus to 186,000 healthy people who had never smoked, however, the relationship between excess weight and early death was more striking. Much as chronic illness confuses the BMI-mortality relationship, the NCI researchers noted, smoking can reduce weight while boosting the risk of death. This study group was large enough to be able to "tease out" the effects of smoking, giving a truer picture of the effects of weight alone.

As a strategy to reduce the distorting effects of pre-existing disease on the relation between excess weight and risk of death, the researchers next analyzed BMI recalled by participants at age 50. This measure represents weight prior to onset of chronic disease, which often leads to weight loss. Among the group of healthy non-smokers, being overweight at age 50 was associated with a 20% to 40% increase in risk of death. Those who were obese saw their risk of death double or triple compared to people of normal weight.

Another prospective study, published in the same issue of the *Journal*, followed 1.2 million Koreans, ages 30 to 95, over a 12-year period. Some 82,000 subjects died during that span. The researchers, at Yonsei University in Korea and Johns Hopkins Bloomberg School of Public Health in Baltimore, found that the risk of death from any cause was lowest among those with a BMI of 23.0 to 24.9. "Underweight, overweight and obese men and women had higher rates of death than men and women of normal weight," concluded lead author Sun Ha Jae, PhD.

The relative risk of death from atherosclerotic cardiovascular disease and cancer was higher among subjects with a greater BMI in the Korean study. Those with a lower BMI, however, were at greater risk of death from respiratory causes. The relationship between BMI and risk of death decreased with advancing age, which is consistent with previous findings that the "ideal" BMI increases with age (see next page).

Bottom line: Normal is best

In an accompanying commentary, Tim Byers, MD, of the University of Colorado School of Medicine pointed out that the Korean study found an increased risk of death even from levels of excess weight that would be considered modest in the US. The two studies spotlight the importance of even small steps to combat weight gain, Dr. Byers said, adding, "Fortunately, evidence points to a substantial health benefit from even small changes in weight trajectory."

Eliseo Guallar, MD, DrPH, a Johns Hopkins professor of epidemiology and co-author of the Korean study, told *The New York Times* that the findings emphasized the importance of maintaining weight in what is considered the "normal" range. He said, "That will help control a whole bunch of other problems."

As for the weight debate, Dr. Leitzmann said, "No single study is able to solve a controversy of this magnitude." But anyone who's overweight, he said, "should be looking to lose weight."

To learn more: *New England Journal of Medicine*, Aug. 24, 2006; abstracts at <content.nejm.org/cgi/content/short/355/8/763>, <content.nejm.org/cgi/content/short/355/8/779>.

BMI Faulted as Obesity Gauge

Even as researchers seem to be confirming the link between abnormal weight and risk of death (see pervious section), two other new studies cast doubt on the most common measure of overweight, obesity and underweight: Body Mass Index (BMI).

Despite the popularity of BMI as a gauge of weight in relationship to height, it's actually not too surprising that it's an imperfect tool, at best. A few years ago, a study hit the headlines proclaiming that most pro football players were overweight or obese, at least judging by their BMI. That's because BMI doesn't differentiate between body fat and muscle mass. Other studies have shown that as you age, a slightly higher BMI serves as a cushion against frailty and chronic disease. And BMI fails to account for the *location* of body fat, whereas studies have shown that abdominal fat tends to be most strongly associated with cardiovascular and other risks.

Those factors may help explain the results of a new Mayo Clinic meta-analysis of 40 studies of 250,152 patients with coronary

Moving Target

Your "ideal BMI"–the figure associated with the lowest risk of chronic disease or mortality–changes with age:

Age range	Male	Female
20-29	21.4	19.5
30-39	21.6	23.4
40-49	22.9	23.2
50-59	25.8	25.2
60-69	26.6	27.3
70-79	27.0	27.8

Behind BMI

Body Mass Index was invented in the 19th century by Adolphe Quetelet, a Belgian statistician and astronomer. In the metric system, BMI is simply weight in kilograms divided by height in meters squared. For US measurements, divide your weight in pounds by your height in inches squared, then multiply by a conversion factor of 703. Or just use one of the many handy BMI calculators online, such as the one at <www.nhlbisupport.com/bmi>. Here are the official definitions:

BMI	Weight Status
Below 18.5	Underweight
18.5-24.9	Normal
25.0-29.9	Overweight
30.0 and Above	Obese

artery disease. The analysis, published in *The Lancet,* found that outcomes for cardiovascular and overall mortality were actually better for overweight and even mildly obese patients than for those with normal BMI.

"Rather than proving that obesity is harmless," study author Francisco Lopez-Jimenez, MD, explained, "our data suggest that alternative methods might be needed to better characterize individuals who truly have excess fat, compared with those in whom BMI is raised because of preserved muscle mass."

Another possible factor, scientists speculated, was that people with low and normal BMI were less likely to get secondary prevention therapies, such as exercise, diet and treatment for other risk factors. Those with BMIs below the "overweight" threshold were less likely to display other known cardiovascular risk factors—so they wouldn't be targets for preventive measures.

In a second BMI study, British researchers followed 14,833 people over age 75 for six years, during which 6,649 died. After adjusting for other factors, they concluded that in this older population, high BMI was not linked to increased risk of death from all causes. Nor was high BMI linked to a greater risk of death from individual causes including circulatory disease, respiratory disease or cancer.

A more accurate predictor of mortality risk, the researchers concluded, was waist-to-hip ratio. That ratio is determined simply by dividing your waist measurement by your hip measurement. Among the over-75 subjects, those with the highest waist-to-hip ratio (closest to 1.0) were 40% more likely to die of cardiovascular disease than those with the lowest ratio (about 0.8).

Senior author Astrid E. Fletcher, MD, a professor of epidemiology at the London School of Hygiene and Tropical Medicine, notes that a low BMI is less desirable in older people because it may indicate poor nutrition or frailty caused by loss of muscle: "The use of BMI is particularly problematic in old age as an indicator of adiposity."

The study, published in the *American Journal of Clinical Nutrition,* found that men with BMI below 23 and women with BMI below 22.3 were actually at highest risk of death.

So is BMI headed for science's trash heap? In a commentary in *The Lancet*, Maria G. Franzosi, MD, of the Istituto Mario Negri in Italy, wasn't quite ready to go that far. But she did conclude, "BMI can definitely be left aside as a clinical and epidemiological measure of cardiovascular risk for both primary and secondary prevention.... BMI is not a good measure of visceral fat, the key determinant of metabolic abnormalities that contribute to cardiovascular risk."

She added that a previous 52-nation study had found the best predictor of heart-attack risk was not BMI but waist-to-hip ratio.

But don't take the doubts about BMI as a license to lose your bathroom scale. Dr. Franzosi cautioned: "Uncertainty about the best index of obesity should not translate into uncertainty about the need for a prevention policy against excess body weight."

Waist-to-Hip Ratio Predicts Heart Risk Better Than BMI

Want a quick assessment of your risk for heart disease? Get out the tape measure.

Researchers at McMaster University near Toronto have found that the best predictor of cardiovascular disease is not Body Mass Index (BMI), the commonly used ratio of weight to height, but rather your waist measurement divided by your hip measurement. A 36-inch waist and 40-inch hips would be a ratio of 0.9, for instance. Anything over 0.85 for women and 0.9 for men indicates greater risk for heart disease. The risk increases continuously with higher waist-to-hip ratio: Those in the highest fifth of people studied were 2.52 times more likely to have a heart attack as those in the lowest fifth.

The researchers analyzed data from the Interheart study of people in 52 countries, comparing 12,461 people who'd suffered a heart attack with 14,637 people free of heart disease. They found that large waist size—indicating dangerous abdominal fat—was harmful, while a larger hip size, possibly indicating lower-body muscle, was protective.

Waist-to-hip ratio was three times more effective than BMI in predicting cardiovascular risk. Previous studies have noted that BMI fails to take into account the location of fat or how muscular a person is—so, for example, more than half of NFL players would be classified as obese. An otherwise skinny person with a potbelly actually is at greater risk of heart disease than someone with a high BMI.

The study reinforces "the whole apple-shaped, pear-shaped thing," according to study co-author Arya Sharma, MD. "What's new here is that BMI falls right out of the equation."

To learn more: *The Lancet*, Nov. 5, 2005. Free abstract online at <www.-thelancet.com/journals/ lancet/issue?volume=366 &issue=9497>.

To learn more: *The Lancet*, Aug. 19; abstract at
<www.thelancet.com/journals/lancet/article/PIIS0140673606692519/abstract>.
American Journal of Clinical Nutrition, August 2006; abstract at
<www.ajcn.org/cgi/content/abstract/84/2/449>.

Go Ahead, Fill Up–But Pick "Low-Energy-Density" Foods

Can you eat more food than most Americans but still consume fewer calories—while getting plenty of key nutrients? Researchers at Penn State University say the answer is yes, as long as you emphasize "low-energy-density" foods. These foods—such as fruits, vegetables and high-fiber grains—have greater volume and so tend to fill you up more, but pack fewer calories per ounce than sugary or fatty foods such as soda pop or snacks.

The new study, published in the *Journal of the American Dietetic Association*, found that people following a low-energy-density diet actually ate more food, by weight, than others in the study group. But those who filled up on fruits, vegetables and fiber consumed fewer calories—an average of 425 fewer for men, 250 fewer for women—and less fat. That low-energy-density group, however, had higher intakes of several important micronutrients, including vitamins A, C and B6, folate, iron, calcium and potassium.

The researchers examined dietary information on 7,500 US adults collected in the 1994-1996 Continuing Survey of Food Intakes by Individuals. They divided the participants into three groups, based on reported food intake: those consuming a low-energy-density diet, medium-energy-density diet and high-energy-density diet.

"These analyses further demonstrate the beneficial effects of a low-energy-density diet, which was associated with lower energy intakes, higher food intakes and higher diet quality than a high-energy-density diet," according to lead researcher Jenny H. Ledikwe, PhD. "To achieve a low-energy-density diet, individuals should be encouraged to eat a variety of fruits and vegetables as well as low-fat/reduced-fat, nutrient-dense, and/or water-rich grains, dairy products, and meats/meat alternatives."

Some previous studies have suggested that reducing calorie density may be a more effective weight-control strategy than concentrating on smaller portion sizes. When people see a packed plate and feel full after a meal, they may not even feel as though they are dieting—despite consuming fewer calories.

To learn more: Journal of the American Dietetic Association, August 2006; abstract at <www.adajournal.org/article/ PIIS0002822306008893/abstract>.

Don't Be Dense!

Tips for reducing your diet's energy density:

- Eat a large salad before the rest of your meal, to fill up on greens (but watch the fatty salad dressings!).

- Change the proportions on your plate, giving more space to vegetables and whole grains and shrinking the space for meat.

- Substitute low-fat dairy foods, lean meat and fish for cheese and fattier cuts.

- Drink water and other non-caloric beverages instead of soda pop and other sugar-sweetened drinks.

- Look for foods high in water and/or fiber content, but low in sugar and fat.

Lose Weight and Chew Gum at the Same Time?

If you need a little help with your New Year's resolution to lose weight in 2006, try reaching for a stick of chewing gum. A new study from the University of Liverpool in England, presented at the annual meeting of the North American Association for the Study of Obesity, suggests that chewing gum can fight the craving for sweets and help suppress your appetite.

The study—which was supported by the Wrigley gum company—involved 60 men and women, ages 18 to 40, whose Body Mass Index (BMI) ranged from a lean 17 to an obese 33. Researchers tested the effect of gum-chewing on post-lunch appetite and afternoon snacking by comparing participants' snack consumption with and without pre-snack chewing gum. On the days when participants chewed gum, they averaged 36 fewer calories from their snack choices. That would add up to 252 fewer calories a week. Subjects' ratings of their afternoon hunger level were also significantly lower when they'd chewed gum. The gum seemed more effective in curbing the desire for sweet snacks than salty treats.

While most of the gum used in the study was sugar-free, even chewing sugary gum wouldn't entirely negate the calorie savings. A stick of regular gum contains about 10 calories, compared to one to three for sugar-free chews.

To learn more: North American Association for the Study of Obesity <www.naaso.org>.

Long-Term Weight Loss:
Six Keys to Keeping It Off

It's a familiar problem: Following this or that diet program, you manage to lose those unwanted 10 pounds. Just months later, though, the scale and your favorite jeans tell you that those 10 pounds are back, maybe with an additional five more. Called "yo-yo dieting" or "weight cycling," it's a common frustration for dieters. With clear links between being obese or overweight and serious illness—including diabetes, stroke and heart disease—it's also dangerous to your health.

But a report on research into long-term weight maintenance offers encouraging news for those ready to leave "fad diets" behind and make more lasting changes. In the report, published in the *American Journal of Clinical Nutrition*, Rena Wing, PhD, a professor at Brown Medical School and director of the Weight Control & Diabetes Research Center at the Miriam Hospital, analyzes the National Weight Control Registry (NWCR), a compilation of individuals who have successfully maintained weight loss.

Funded in part by the National Institutes of Health, the NWCR is a different kind of study. Rather than randomly putting people into groups and testing weight-loss methods, researchers set up a registry open to anyone who's lost at least 30 pounds and kept it off at least one year. Those who enroll fill out questionnaires about how they lost weight, how they're trying to keep it off and other aspects of their health. More than 6,000 success stories have signed up to date.

The average weight lost by participants is nearly 73 pounds, and that loss has been maintained over an average six years. Of the group, 77% are women, 82% are college educated, 95% are Caucasian and 64% are married. Average age at entry is nearly 47.

Registrants reported using a variety of diets, exercise and behavioral changes to lose weight. But while weight-loss techniques varied, some common techniques and habits for keeping the weight off emerged.

Wing identified six successful practices for long-term weight maintenance:

1. Engage in physical activity. More than 90% of those who've kept their weight off use physical activity as part of their weight-control program. While only 1% of the NWCR group used exercise alone to achieve and maintain their weight loss, experts agree that increased activity, along with a healthy diet, is a key component of any successful weight program.

The flip side of physical activity is not being a "couch potato." Almost two-thirds of those in the registry watch less than 10 hours of TV per week—much less than the national average. (If you can't tune out, try mild exercise—instead of eating!—while you watch.)

2. Eat a low-calorie, low-fat diet. NWCR participants reported they consumed, on average, only 24% of their calories from fat. And watch the fast food: People in the registry eat fast food less than once a week, and eat out at restaurants of any kind no more than three times a week.

The math is simple: To keep from gaining weight, your calorie intake must not exceed the calories you burn.

Twice as many participants, nearly 88%, relied on careful food selection as opposed to restricting the amount and types of food they ate. Making healthy choices from a wide variety of foods proved to be effective for weight loss and maintenance, perhaps in part because such regimens are easier to adhere to over the long haul.

3. Eat breakfast regularly. Breakfast helps controls hunger and prevent binge eating later in the day.

4. Maintain a consistent eating pattern across weekdays and weekends. Those who "go off their diet" on weekends, vacations or holidays have a harder time keeping weight off.

5. Self-monitor your weight. Weigh yourself daily, NWCR experts advise.

6. Catch "slips" before they turn into larger weight regains. Plan for how to get back on track if your weight begins to creep up.

An analysis of NCWR experiences also suggests weight-loss maintenance may get easier over time. After individuals successfully maintained

---

Smarter Snacking

The American Heart Association suggests eating these healthy snacks to avoid hunger, overeating at meals and splurging on high-calorie snacks. Remember to watch out for "added calories"–don't sweeten beverages, or stick to no-calorie sweetener if you do. Watch sodium content in drinks and soups.

Keep some healthy snacks–things you'll enjoy grabbing–in the house at all times, in your desk at work, and in your purse or briefcase. Then when hunger strikes, you can "quiet the beast" with something healthy.

- **Munchies:** a whole grain piece of bread with a thin slice of part-skim mozzarella cheese; plain low-fat yogurt; plain, unbuttered popcorn; rice cakes; a few almonds or walnuts
- **Crunchies:** apples and pears; carrot and celery sticks; green pepper strips; zucchini slices; radishes; broccoli spears; cauliflowerettes
- **Hot drinks:** clear soups, such as broth; vegetable or tomato soup; hot tea; heated skim milk with a little cocoa in it
- **Thirst quenchers:** skim milk; unsweetened juices; tomato or mixed vegetable juice; ice water garnished with a twist of lemon or lime
- **For a sweet tooth:** canned fruit in its natural juice, not syrup; a thin slice of angel food cake; a baked apple; a cup of sugar-free gelatin

their weight loss for two to five years, the odds of longer-term success greatly increased.

Robin B. Kanarek, PhD, professor of nutrition and behavior at Tufts' Friedman School of Nutrition Science and Policy, agrees that small, consistent behavioral changes can help individuals lose weight and maintain the loss. Rather than making abrupt or drastic changes in diet or behavior patterns, Kanarek says individuals can make simple, healthy changes that lead to substantial reductions in body weight.

Becoming aware of what you're actually consuming is the first step to identifying unhealthy dietary habits, such as a diet high in fat or a pattern of consuming frequent high-calorie snacks. Simply writing down what you eat leads to weight loss in most individuals, according to Kanarek.

Next, pay attention to portion size. In a restaurant, take a moment to assess how much is on the plate—has it been "super-sized"? Often you can be satisfied with half of what is served, taking the leftovers home. If you want

---

Smarter Snacking
The Facts on Five Diet Myths

Though we all "ought" to know better, the desire for quick weight loss often tempts us into unhealthy practices, the results of which are almost always temporary. Have you fallen prey to any of these popular dieting myths, identified and "busted" by the Weight-control Information Network of the National Institute of Diabetes and Digestive and Kidney Diseases?

Myth: Fad diets work for permanent weight loss.

Fact: Fad diets often promise quick weight loss or tell you to cut certain foods out of your diet. Diets that strictly limit calories or food choices are hard to follow, and most people quickly tire of them. You may lose weight at first on one of these diets, but then regain the pounds, and often more.

Fad diets may be unhealthy because they may not provide all the nutrients your body needs. Also, losing weight at a very rapid rate (more than three pounds a week after the first couple of weeks) may increase your risk for developing gallstones. Diets providing fewer than 800 calories per day can result in heart rhythm abnormalities, which can be fatal.

Tip: Research suggests that losing up to two pounds a week by making healthy food choices, eating moderate portions, and building physical activity into your daily life is the best way to lose weight and keep it off. By adopting healthy eating and physical activity habits, you may also lower your risk for developing type 2 diabetes, heart disease and high blood pressure.

Myth: High-protein/low-carbohydrate diets are a healthy way to lose weight.

Fact: The long-term health effects of a high-protein/low carbohydrate diet are unknown, but common sense tells us that getting most of our daily calories from high-protein foods like meat, eggs and cheese is not a balanced eating plan. You may be eating too much saturated fat and cholesterol, which can raise heart-disease risk. You may be eating too few fruits, vegetables and whole grains, which can lead to constipation due to lack of dietary fiber. Following a high-protein/low-carbohydrate diet may also make you feel nauseous, tired and weak. Eating fewer than 130 grams of carbohydrate a day can lead to a dangerous buildup of ketones in the blood.

Tip: A reduced-calorie eating plan that includes recommended amounts of carbohydrates, protein and fat will allow you to lose weight in a healthy, sustainable manner.

Myth: Starches are fattening and should be limited when trying to lose weight.

Fact: Many foods high in starch, such as bread, rice, pasta, cereals, beans, fruits and some vegetables (like potatoes and yams) are low in fat and calories. They become high in fat and calories when eaten in large portion sizes or when covered with high-fat toppings like butter, sour cream or mayonnaise. Some foods high in starch—complex carbohydrates—are an important source of energy for your body.

Tip: The Dietary Guidelines for Americans recommends eating 6 to 11 servings a day, depending on your calorie needs, from the bread, cereal, rice and pasta group—even when trying to lose weight. Pay attention to your serving sizes, and pick whole grains over processed grains. Choose other starchy foods that are high in dietary fiber, too, such as beans, peas and other vegetables.

Myth: Certain foods, like grapefruit, celery or cabbage soup, can burn fat and make you lose weight.

Fact: No foods can burn fat. Some foods with caffeine may speed up your metabolism (the way your body burns calories) for a short time, but they do not cause weight loss.

Tip: The best way to lose weight is to cut back on the number of calories you eat and be more physically active.

Myth: Natural or herbal weight-loss products are safe and effective.

Fact: A weight-loss product that claims to be "natural" or "herbal" is not necessarily safe. These products are seldom scientifically tested to prove that they are safe or that they work. For example, herbal products containing ephedra (now banned by the US government) have caused serious health problems and even death. Newer products that claim to be ephedra-free are not necessarily danger-free, because they may contain ingredients similar to ephedra.

Tip: Talk with your health-care provider before using any weight-loss product.

To learn more: National Institute of Diabetes and Digestive and Kidney Diseases
<win.niddk.nih.gov/publications/myths.htm>.

dessert, skip the appetizer, bread or salad.

To learn more: *American Journal of Clinical Nutrition,* July 2005, <www.ajcn.org>. National Weight Control Registry <www.nwcr.ws>.

Watch Your Weight to Beat Heartburn & Reflux

Bothered by persistent heartburn or acid reflux—the painful symptoms of gastroesophageal reflux disease (GERD), which is caused by stomach acids backing up into your esophagus? Relief may be as close as your bathroom scale.

Shedding extra pounds can reduce a woman's risk of heartburn by as much as 40%, according to new Nurses' Health Study research published in the *New England Journal of Medicine.* On the other hand, while previous research has shown a link between GERD and overweight or obesity, the study also found that even moderate weight gain can double the risk of heartburn and acid reflux.

The study looked at GERD symptoms and changes in body-mass index (BMI) over a span of 14 years, in women of normal weight as well as in overweight women. It used data on 10,545 participants in the long-running Nurses' Health Study, 22% of whom reported suffering GERD symptoms at least weekly; regardless of frequency, 3,419 of the women described their symptoms as moderately severe.

"Finding such a direct and strong link between heartburn and BMI was

Heartburn, American Style

Is heartburn mostly a phenomenon of Western culture–and our supersized, cheeseburger-laden eating patterns? That's the suggstion of a review of 31 published studies on gastroesophageal reflux disease (GERD), encompassing data on 77,671 patients. The review, by Paul Moayyedi, MD, of the Mayo Clinic and Nicholas J. Talley, MD, of McMaster University Medical Center, found that heartburn is much less common in east Asian countries than in the US. Compared to Americans, only about one-third as many Asian people suffer weekly heartburn, and only half as many have symptoms at least once a month. The review couldn't pinpoint why we're more likely to suffer heartburn, but cited several possible lifestyle factors as well as heredity (which may account for 31%-43% of GERD cases).

To learn more: *The Lancet,* June 24, 2006.

really striking," says the study's lead author, Brian C. Jacobson, MD, MPH, of Boston University Medical Center. "If you have heartburn and have put on weight, even if you are not overweight, your heartburn could be due to the additional pounds. If you lose weight, your symptoms likely will improve."

The study found the risk of frequent GERD symptoms, such as heartburn and acid reflux, rose progressively with increasing BMI. Compared to women with a BMI of 20-22.4, the risk was only two-thirds as high for those with a BMI under 20. But that comparative GERD risk jumped to 38% higher for BMI of 22.5-24.9—still considered normal weight. For overweight women, defined as a BMI of 25-29.9, the risk of frequent GERD symptoms was more than double. And for obese women, with a BMI of 30-plus, the risk soared to nearly triple.

Even modest weight gain could cause or exacerbate GERD symptoms. In women with a normal baseline BMI (between 18.5 and 24.9), an increase

I'm OK, You're Fat

We know our fellow Americans are too fat–but we don't seem able to see our own obesity in the mirror. That's the conclusion of a Pew Research Center telephone survey that found 90% of Americans are aware of what's been called the "obesity epidemic." Those same respondents, however, reported their own height and weight both taller and slimmer than the actual US average. Men in particular gave themselves two inches of "phantom height" (5-foot-11 versus the actual US median 5-foot-9), lessening the waistline impact of their weight.

Nationally, almost two-thirds of adults are obese or overweight, and indeed 70% of respondents to the Pew survey agreed that most of the people they know are too heavy. But only 39% of respondents confessed that they themselves were even "a little" overweight. When Americans think about weight, the Pew report concludes, "they appear to use different scales for different people."

To learn more: "American See Weight Problems Everywhere But in the Mirror," online at <pewresearch.org/assets/social/pdf/Obesity.pdf>.

in BMI of more than 3.5 was associated with a significantly increased risk of frequent GERD symptoms. For a 5-foot-6-inch woman who weighs 125 pounds, an increase of 22 pounds would boost her BMI by 3.5 points, from 20.2 to 23.7.

GERD affects up to 60% of the population at some point over the span of a year, and 20-30% suffer at least weekly. Its painful symptoms lead to some 9 million doctor visits annually in the US, at a treatment cost of about $10 billion a year. Even more seriously, acid reflux has been linked to esophageal cancer, the incidence of which has been increasing as the population has grown more overweight.

Dr. Jacobson, who says he plans to study whether the same relationship between BMI and GERD holds for men, says that the results of the study are of particular concern given increasing rates of obesity. "As a nation we are getting heavier, which means the probability of heartburn will only get worse," he says. "Each year we spend billions of dollars on treating heartburn, and this study suggests we will only be spending more and more."

To learn more: *New England Journal of Medicine,* June 1, 2006; abstract at <content.nejm.org/cgi/ content/abstract/354/ 22/2340>.
Free BMI calculator at <www.nhlbisupport.com/bmi>.

How Eating Out Adds Up

If you're watching your waistline, don't lose focus just because somebody else is preparing the food. Americans are eating out more than ever, which may be one reason more than 65% of us are now overweight or obese. According to a new report by The Keystone Center, commissioned by the US Food and Drug Administration (FDA), Americans spend about 46% of their food budget on food prepared away from home and take in 32% of their calories from restaurant or takeout foods. The report urges restaurants to enlist in the fight against obesity by shrinking portion sizes, emphasizing more fruits and vegetables in their menus, and listing the calorie count for menu items. The most popular menu choices when Americans eat out? According to a 2005 report by The NPD Group, our top picks are hamburgers, French fries and pizza.

To learn more: Keystone Forum on Away-from-Home Foods <www.keystone.org/spp/ documents/ Forum_Report_FINAL_5-30-06.pdf>.

The US Weighs In

Globally speaking, the US is pulling its own weight—and then some. An *American Demographics* analysis of World Health Organization data on the 25 most populous nations says the US has nearly 23% of the world's obese population age 15 and up (versus just 4.6% of the total global population). We've got barely more than our share—7%—of the merely overweight. But the, er, heavy preponderance of obese Americans pushes the US' average body mass index (BMI) to 28.4 for men and 28.8 for women, versus global averages of 24.4 and 25.3, respectively. The average American male, age 20-74, now weighs 191 pounds, while females weigh in at 164.3 pounds—both figures up more than 24 pounds since the early 1960s. We lead the world with 74.1% overweight or obese, compared to a 34.5% global average and well ahead of runnersup Egypt (69.3%), Mexico (68.1%), the United Kingdom (63.8%) and Germany (60%). And there may be something to that title, French Women Don't Get Fat: France ranks below most other European nations, with 40% obese or overweight. Among industrialized nations where famine is not a greater concern than overeating, Japan stands the skinniest, with 22.4% obese or overweight.

To learn more: *American Demographics* <adage.com/americandemographics/
article?article_id=109172>.

49 States Loosening Belts

Only one state—Nevada—managed to decrease its percentage of obese adults last year, according to an annual report by the Trust for America's Health. Nationwide, the report found waistlines continuing to expand, with obesity now exceeding 25% in 13 states. The state with the highest proportion of obese citizens remains Mississippi, at 29.5%—up 1.1% from the year before. Colorado is still the leanest state, virtually unchanged at 16.9% obese.

Janet Collins, MD, of the Centers for Disease Control noted the connection between poverty and obesity. The five states with the greatest obesity problem—Mississippi, Alabama, West Virginia, Louisiana and Kentucky—all also suffer poverty rates higher than the national average.

To learn more: Trust for America's Health <healthyamericans.org>.

Getting in Shape, the Smart Way

9 Easy Ways to Add Exercise to Every Day

Research has shown that exercise can add not only years to your life, but life to your years, improving flexibility and balance while combating conditions ranging from diabetes to maybe even Alzheimer's disease. Studies have shown that exercise and diet combined are more effective in helping reach weight-loss goals than diet alone, and that there's nothing as effective as regular exercise to keep weight off. So why do so many of us find it so hard to get off the couch and onto the treadmill?

Rebecca Seguin, MS, CSCS, project manager at the Center for Physical Activity & Nutrition in Tufts' Friedman School, says that even among retirees, finding time to work out is a commonly cited obstacle to getting on and sticking with a program of regular physical activity. Getting past that obstacle and adding some form of regular exercise to our daily lives is crucial, she says.

"Many of the things we think of as related to aging are really related to a loss of muscle mass and strength over time," Seguin says. "And it can have a 'snowball effect.' People suffer incremental losses over a period of time and this eventually leads to weakness, loss of balance, and ultimately a loss of independence."

Seguin has co-authored a book, *Growing Stronger,* produced through a three-year grant and collaboration with the Center for Disease Control and published by Tufts, designed to help older adults improve their health through an easily implemented, mostly home-based program of regular exercise.

"Walking is a great place to start," Seguin says, "but it doesn't help us hold onto our muscle mass. Starting around midlife, we lose up to a quarter to a third of a pound of muscle mass per year if we don't do anything to prevent it. That adds up! Strength training, lifting weights, is what helps us maintain—or regain—our muscular strength and bone mass."

Acceptance of where you are and establishing a realistic program you can follow, Seguin says, is the first step. "Start out without any weights, just to get moving," she says. "I absolutely recommend trying to find a group to exercise with if at all possible, particularly for those who have had trouble sticking with a program. The social aspect alone can keep them coming back."

And there's good news for the "chronically busy": Many things you might not think of as exercise are considered "moderate level" physical activities. The simple movements involved in performing daily chores can add up—boosting heart rate, burning calories and strengthening muscle groups. Employed in a deliberate, focused way, these everyday tasks could be the perfect way to start getting back in shape.

Exercise physiologists define "moderate activity" as anything that raises your body to three to six times your average resting metabolic rate (expressed in units called metabolic equivalents, or METs). Depending on size, your body at rest burns around 70 calories an hour on average. So three METs is equal to expending approximately 210 calories. You need to expend three to six METs over a period of 30 minutes, five to seven days a week, to gain significant health benefits. Most household activities take three to four METs to perform.

Try these nine ideas to start making exercise part of your daily routine. While not all of them will always qualify as "moderate activity," all nine will help get you in the habit of upping your activity level whenever possible:

1.Take the scenic route.

Walking is a great way to get exercise, requires no special equipment beyond a decent pair of shoes or sneakers, and can be practiced pretty much anywhere and anytime. There are many creative ways to add steps to your day. Park farther from your destination—the grocery store, mall, post office—any time you can and it is safe to do so.

At the grocery store, take a walk around the entire store before you actually begin to shop, making note of the things you need and special items or sales. If you go out for lunch, walk to your destination if possible, and take a longer and different route back home, for variety and the extra steps. Casual walking takes up to 3.5 METs and burns about 245 calories per hour.

2.Get swept away.

Vacuuming, sweeping and raking all involve your arm and leg muscles and expend up to four METs per hour, burning 245-280 calories an hour. By vacuuming for 10 minutes, sweeping the sidewalk for 10 minutes and raking the yard for 10 minutes, you add a half-hour of moderate physical activity to your day.

3.Get dancing.

Take a class in ballroom, salsa or swing dancing. You'll have fun in a new social setting while getting a low-impact aerobic workout. Dancing expends about 4.5 METs per hour, more if you really "hoof it," and burns upwards of 315 calories.

Shy? Turn on the radio or put on your favorite CD and dance with abandon in the privacy of your own home.

The Arthritis Foundation recommends dancing as a form of exercise for people with fibromyalgia, as it employs smooth, dynamic movements rather than tightening one particular muscle, which can cause soreness.

4. Make TV time "active time."

Jog lightly in place or do floor exercise on a yoga mat while you watch TV. If you have a stationary bike or treadmill, put it in front of the TV and work out while you watch your favorite show. Do leg lifts with ankle weights or arm curls with dumbbells. Such exercise can use up to eight METs and burn 550 calories or more per hour while toning and strengthening leg and/or arm muscles.

Leg lifts strain your back? Sit in a solid chair and lift one leg slowly until it's parallel with the floor. Hold for a few seconds, then slowly lower it. Do some lifts with your toes pointed away from you and some with your toes pointed toward you to work different muscles. Then repeat with the other leg. As you get used to the activity, increase repetitions, then add ankle weights.

5. Dig in.

Gardening and other routine yardwork activities help strengthen knees, arms and hands. Pulling weeds, mowing and raking involve the back, arm and leg muscles. Such activities can burn 300 calories per hour—and get you out in the fresh air.

6. Hop to it.

Do 5-10 minutes of jumping jacks. They're fun, encourage balance and flexibility, and can burn 90 calories in one 10-minute session.

7. Turn up the heat while cooking.

Do standing push-ups while you wait for a pot to boil. Stand about an arm's length from the kitchen counter, and push your arms against the counter. Push in and out to work your arms and shoulders.

8.Make nap time "your time."

If you're housebound, caring for a sick loved one, hop on an exercise bike or treadmill while your ailing charge naps.

9. Fill your waiting time.

If you're waiting for an elevator or on hold on the telephone, work your abdominal muscles: Stand with your feet parallel and your knees relaxed. Contract the muscles around your belly button. Then elevate your upper torso, and release. Finally, contract your buttocks for a few seconds.

While waiting at the bathroom sink for a facial or hair-color process, do arm curls with small dumbbells. Keep a set of small weights handy by the sink.

Waiting for the doctor? Ask the receptionist for an estimate on your wait time, then take a brisk walk around the building. You'll get fresh air and add steps to your day, and the time may even seem to pass more quickly!

If you're waiting for a child or grandchild to take a music lesson or practice sports, use the time to take a brisk walk.

To learn more: To order the *Growing Stronger* book on strength training for older adults, go to <www.healthletter.tufts.edu>. An interactive program based on the book is online at <nutrition.tufts.edu/ research/growingstronger>.

Stick With It

If you find your commitment to your exercise program lagging, consider these suggestions to help you stay on the path to fitness:

Have fun: Enjoying your workout will increase the odds that you'll keep at it. Join in group sports or physical activities like swimming or yoga that suit your personality.

Be conscious of your motivation: Research shows that people who have positive personal goals for their exercise regimen are more likely to develop and stick with a healthy routine than those who think of exercise as something they "should do."

Reward yourself: Associating exercise with something pleasant can encourage commitment. Schedule your workouts right before something you enjoy, like a favorite television program. Allow yourself time to read the paper and enjoy breakfast after a morning workout, or soak in a luxurious bath after your evening session.

Accept and adjust: Set safe and realistic goals for yourself, and set yourself up to succeed. Talk with your health professional, especially if you have physical limitations like arthritis or a heart condition. Be willing to adjust your goals and routine. If swimming isn't working out for you, try something else, like a Tai Chi class or stationary bike.

Make it convenient: Studies show that people are more likely to continue with an exercise program when there's not a lot of hassle involved. Choose a gym or walking trail near your house. Consider buying exercise equipment for your home and set it up in an area that's easily accessible and that you'll like to spend time in.

Mix it up: Varying your routine will ensure that you have another activity to enjoy—maybe yoga, cycling or dance—when you're not in the mood to lift weights, for instance.

Schedule it: You're more likely to follow through with an exercise routine when you're deliberate about your commitment. Write it down! You're more likely to make the time and space for your workout when it's on your calendar. Find a time of day that works for you.

Track your progress: Research shows that people who stick with their exercise regimen for six months are more likely to make increased activity a healthy habit for life. Keep a journal of your progress, mark off your achievements on your calendar, or keep track online at sites such as <www.nutrition.tufts.edu/research/growingstronger> or <www.justmove.org>.

Consider a trainer: A personal trainer or fitness coach can customize a program to your goals and needs, and ensure your safety during workouts.

Lifting Weights Attacks Unhealthy Belly Fat in Women

Hitting the weight room twice a week for an hour can help women prevent or at least slow "middle-aged spread," the onerous buildup of tummy fat that often takes hold with aging, a new study suggests. And that's good news since belly fat—the deep fat that wraps itself around organs—is linked with heart disease and other ailments.

"On average, women in the middle years of their lives gain one to two pounds a year, and most of this is assumed to be fat," says study lead author Kathryn H. Schmitz, PhD, assistant professor at the University of Pennsylvania's Center for Clinical Epidemiology and Biostatistics. "This study shows that strength training can prevent increases in body fat percentage and attenuate increases in the fat deposit most closely associated with heart disease."

The study, funded by the National Institutes of Health and recently presented at an American Heart Association conference, evenly divided 164 overweight and obese Minnesota women, ages 24 to 44, into two groups. One group participated in a two-year weight-training program, while the others were simply given a brochure recommending exercise of 30 minutes to an hour most days of the week. Both groups were told not to change their diets in a way that might lead to weight changes.

Using both free weights and machines, the women in the strength-training group worked out for about an hour in supervised classes, focusing on the chest, back, shoulders, biceps, triceps, lower back, buttocks and thigh areas, and were encouraged to gradually increase the weights they lifted.

Women who did the weight-training for two years decreased their overall body fat percentage by almost 4%, while the group just given advice remained the same. Even more significantly, the strength-training group saw only a 7% increase in intra-abdominal fat, where the advice-only group experienced a 21% increase.

Need more motivation to lose that abdominal flab? Researchers have shown that belly fat has been linked with Type II diabetes, gallstones and shortness of breath.

To learn more: American Heart Association
<www.americanheart.org/presenter.jhtml?identifier=3038032>.

Want to Live Longer? Take a Walk

Getting up off your duff can add almost four years to your life, according to a new analysis of data from the long-running Framingham Heart Study. Although many previous studies have shown a range of health benefits from physical activity—from weight loss to reducing the risk of illness to keeping the mind sharp with aging—this is the first to directly calculate the effect of exercise on lifespan. The major contributor to the more-active subjects' longer lives was a postponing of cardiovascular disease, the nation's number-one killer.

Looking at data on more than 5,200 study participants age 50 and older, the researchers found that men who engaged in moderate physical activity—equivalent to 30 minutes of walking daily, five days a week—lived 1.3 years longer and enjoyed 1.1 more years free of cardiovascular disease. Moderately active women saw similar benefits, living 1.5 years longer, 1.3 years more without cardiovascular disease.

Those who managed a high level of physical activity—equal to running 30 minutes daily, five days a week—significantly extended their lives. Men added 3.7 years in life expectancy, 3.2 years without cardiovascular disease, and women lived an average of 3.5 years longer than their sedentary peers, 3.3 more years free of cardiovascular disease.

Lead author Oscar H. Franco, MD, PhD, of Erasmus MC University Medical Center in the Netherlands, pointed out that not only do the physically active live longer, they also live healthier lives. "Our study suggests that following an active lifestyle is an effective way to achieve healthy aging," Dr. Franco concluded.

The findings were published in the *Archives of Internal Medicine*, along with a second study of sedentary Americans who took up walking. This two-year study randomly assigned 492 adults, ages 30 to 69, to four walking-exercise regimens—combining either moderate or hard intensity exercise with low or high frequency of activity—or a comparison group. Significant improvement in cardiorespiratory fitness was seen in three of the walking groups: those who walked at either moderate or hard intensity for 30 minutes five days a week and those who walked at hard intensity only three to four times a week. Only the high frequency-hard intensity group also showed improvement in cholesterol levels, and these were short-term.

One of the goals of this study, according to principal investigator Michael Perri, PhD, of the University of Florida, was to learn about how people respond to exercise prescriptions on their own, rather than in laboratory settings. "When exercising on their own, people generally complete only about 60% of the amount prescribed," Perri noted. "As a result, an exercise prescription for moderate-intensity walking on three to four days a week may not generate a large enough amount of exercise to produce a change in fitness."

In an editorial in the same issue of the journal, Steven Blair, PhD, of the Cooper Institute concluded, "The bottom line is that 30 minutes of walking on five to seven days a week provides substantial health benefits."

To learn more: *Archives of Internal Medicine,* Nov. 14, 2005. Free abstracts at <archinte.ama-assn.org/cgi/content/abstract/165/20/2355> and <archinte.ama-assn.org/cgi/content/abstract/165/20/2362>.

Fitness Quick Facts

Dog Walking Beats Popular Diets

Want to lose weight? Get a dog. A study by the University of Missouri-Columbia's Research Center for Human-Animal Interaction found that having—and walking—a dog can encourage people to get more exercise and lose more weight than popular diet plans. The human participants, who walked "loaner" dogs for 50 weeks, lost an average of 14 pounds. They began by walking 10 minutes daily, three times a week, working up to a routine of 20 minutes a day, five times a week.

"Many of them told us that they didn't necessarily walk in the study because they knew it was good for their health," says Rebecca Johnson, PhD, RN, an associate professor of nursing and director of the center. "They enjoyed walking because they knew it was good for the animals."

To Learn More: <www.missouri.edu/~nursing/ about/profiles/johnson.php>

Watch Your Steps

Don't scrimp when buying a pedometer–that cheap model might be as much as half off in counting your steps. Researchers at Ghent University in Belgium discovered the downside of bargain pedometers when they planned a large community campaign to get people walking 10,000 steps a day. Before rolling out the program, which was going to use cheap pedometers that could be handed out free, the researchers tested the accuracy of their $1.20 Stepping Meters. So they compared 973 Stepping Meters against the Yamax Digiwalker SW-200 (about $19 in the US), considered the "gold standard" in pedometers for its accuracy and reliability. Only 26% of the cheap pedometers got an acceptable score–defined as no more than a 10% variation in step count from the Digiwalker. More than a third–36.6%–of the Stepping Meters miscounted steps by 50% or more. Although more than two-thirds of the inaccurate counters overestimated the number of steps taken, researchers noted there was no consistency in performance. That means, given a 20% error rate, someone aiming for 10,000 steps daily could actually be walking only 8,000 steps–or as many as 12,000.

To learn more: *British Journal of Sports Medicine,* online first, June 21, 2006; abstract at <bjsm.bmjjournals.com/cgi/content/abstract/ bjsm.2005.025296v1>.

Experts to US: Get Physical!

Two new reports show how Americans have become couch potatoes. The first, issued by the US Centers for Disease Control and Prevention (CDC), found that 54.1% of American adults fail to get the minimum level of physical activity necessary for health benefits—at least a half-hour daily. And 15% of adults are "physically inactive" in all three areas the report examined—household work, transportation and discretionary/leisure time. The statistics did show a small improvement from two years before. But 12 states and territories actually saw declines in activity, with the greatest growth in couch potatoes coming in Florida, North Carolina, West Virginia and Puerto Rico.

The second report, published in the *Journal of the American Medical Association,* suggests that 19% of Americans ages 12 through 49—some 16 million people—are woefully out of shape, unable to pass a basic fitness test. Researchers at Northwestern University studied more than 3,000 adolescents and almost 2,200 adults, all free of cardiovascular disease, using a treadmill to test heart rate and estimated aerobic capacity. They categorized participants as high, moderate and low fitness based on the results. About 14% of the adults landed in the lowest group; alarmingly, nearly 34% of adolescents failed the fitness test. Overall, women were less fit than men. Members of the low-fitness group were more likely to have cardiovascular-disease risk factors, such as being overweight or having newly identified hypertension or high cholesterol. "The correlations we report between low fitness and cardiovascular disease risk factors suggest a potential trend of increasing morbidity and mortality from chronic diseases," the researchers warned, "the first sign of which is the burgeoning obesity epidemic."

To learn more: *Morbidity and Mortality Weekly Report,* Dec. 1, 2005, online at <www.cdc.gov/mmwr/preview/mmwrhtml/ss5408a1.htm>. *Journal of the American Medical Association,* Dec. 21, 2005. Free abstract at <jama.ama-assn.org/cgi/content/short/ 294/23/2981>.

Tune in to Exercise

Can't stick to your exercise routine? Maybe an iPod would help. Research at Fairleigh Dickinson University, presented at the annual conference of NAASO, the Obesity Society, suggests that tuning in to music while exercising helps overweight people stick with it and get better results. The researchers evaluated the effect of music on exercise adherence in 41 moderately obese to overweight women as part of a 24-week weight-loss program. The group that walked to music lost significantly more weight and body fat than those who went tuneless. The music listeners also adhered better to the walking part of the regimen and were less likely to drop out.

To learn more: NAASO, the Obesity Society, <www.naaso.org>.

Exercise Efficiency Can Be Regained

As you get older, you lose "exercise efficiency"—how much energy you need to expend for a given physical activity—but new research suggests it's possible to regain some of that youthful efficiency. Scientists at the University of Washington compared sedentary adults in their 60s and 70s with counterparts in their 20s and 30s, before and after a six-month exercise regimen. Initially, older subjects had to use much more oxygen to maintain the same walking pace as younger participants. After the program of exercising 90 minutes a day, three times a week, however, the older people closed much of that gap: They improved exercise efficiency by 30%, while younger exercisers gained only 2%. Inactivity, researchers concluded, may be largely responsible for the decline in exercise efficiency with age—not the inevitable accumulation of years.

To learn more: *Journal of the American College of Cardiology,* March 7, 2006; free abstract at <dx.doi.org/10.1016/j.jacc.2005.09.066>.

Eating to Beat Heart Disease

Diet Plus Lifestyle Changes Equal Heart Health

The path to heart health starts on your plate—but doesn't stop there. That's the message of new American Heart Association (AHA) guidelines, the first update to its official recommendations in six years. As a sign of the increased focus on physical activity, weight control and avoiding tobacco, the word "lifestyle" was added to the title of the 2006 AHA Diet and Lifestyle Recommendations.

"What's really new is the emphasis on the whole package—not just diet," says Alice Lichtenstein, DSc, Gershoff Professor of nutrition science and policy at Tufts' Friedman School, who chaired the AHA committee that revised the guidelines. "The previous recommendations stressed a healthy dietary pattern; the new ones broaden that concept to include the importance of a healthy lifestyle pattern. The two go together—they should be inseparable."

Shunning fad diets and temporary fixes, the AHA's Nutrition Committee instead urges long-term, permanent changes in how we eat and live. "These are not necessarily major changes," says Lichtenstein. "Small, gradual changes are more likely to be sustained over time." Examples might include switching to low- and non-fat dairy products, she suggests, or opting for brown rice instead of white. "People can continue to eat what they enjoy, but make changes in portion size, or in the proportion of meat to vegetables at dinner."

Similarly, although the guidelines call for 30 minutes of physical activity most days of the week, that doesn't have to mean a solid half-hour on the treadmill. "We don't expect everyone to join a gym or become a jock," says Lichtenstein. "It does not have to be done all at once—accumulating 30 minutes throughout the day is fine—and, of course, more is better. No one is too old or too out of shape to make small changes to increase physical activity."

The bottom line—and this, too, is a fresh emphasis in the updated recommendations—is to balance the calories you eat against those you burn. Says Lichtenstein, "We wanted to address head-on the worsening obesity epidemic, because of the impact of body weight on the risk of cardiovascular disease."

Besides scrutinizing portion sizes—not only at home but also at restaurants—a good first step to controlling intake is to cut back on nutrient-poor foods, such as the "liquid calories" in soft drinks, fruit juices, coffee concoctions and alcoholic beverages. "People don't realize the significant number of calories they get from fluids, and there's research suggesting that such calories may not be as satiating," Lichtenstein says. "That doesn't mean you can't have your orange juice in the morning, but liquid calories can really add up."

More Heart-Healthy Strategies

• Eating a variety of fruits and vegetables helps control weight and blood pressure.

• Unrefined whole-grain foods can lower cholesterol and help you feel "full."

• Choose lean meats and poultry without skin and prepare them without added saturated and trans fat.

• Select fat-free, 1% fat and low-fat dairy products.

• Cut back on beverages and foods with added sugars.

• When eating out, split an entree or order two or three appetizers instead.

• Ask for sauces and dressings on the side.

• Choose foods that have been grilled, baked, steamed or poached.

The AHA recommendations also include specific goals to make diets more heart-healthy:

• Limit saturated fat to less than 7% of calories (down from 10% in the 2000 guidelines).

• Limit trans fat to less than 1% of calories—the AHA's first specific figure on these dangerous fats.

• Aim to eat less than 300 milligrams of cholesterol daily.

• Reduce sodium intake to less than 2,300 milligrams a day.

• Limit alcohol to two drinks a day for men, one for women.

• Eat fish twice a week, especially varieties high in omega-3 fatty acids.

• Eat a diet rich in vegetables, fruits and whole grains, aiming for about 25 grams of fiber daily.

Of the updated recommendations about fats, Lichtenstein explains,

"The point is not to calculate the amount of saturated and trans-fatty acids in the diet, but to choose foods that minimize your intake. For example, you can choose leaner cuts of meat and lower-fat dairy products, smaller serving sizes, avoid foods made with hydrogenated fat and include more fruits, vegetables, vegetarian options and fish in the diet."

The AHA also seeks to enlist the help of health professionals, restaurants, the food industry, schools and government. The recommendations include suggestions for these special audiences, such as displaying caloric content prominently on menus, reducing portion size, limiting trans fatty acids and using low-saturated-fatty-acid oils in food preparation.

To learn more: "Making Healthy Food and Lifestyle Choices" free brochure <www.americanheart.org/ presenter.jhtml?identifier=3040210>.

Five Healthy Lifestyle Factors Fight Heart Disease in Men

Can a heart-healthy lifestyle really make a difference? A new study published in the American Heart Association journal *Circulation* says yes—and that it's never too late to start. Researchers at the Harvard School of Public Health (HSPH) identified five key healthy lifestyle factors, then looked at 42,847 men, ages 40 to 75, over a 16-year period to see how their lifestyles matched up with risk of coronary heart disease (CHD). The study found that even men taking antihypertensive or lipid-lowering medications may reduce their risk of heart problems through lifestyle choices.

The researchers defined these five healthy lifestyle factors:

1. Not smoking

2. Daily exercise (at least 30 minutes)

3. Moderate alcohol consumption (an average of one-half to two drinks daily)

4. A healthy body weight (measured as a Body Mass Index under 25)

5. A healthy diet (based upon the Alternate Healthy Eating Index developed by HSPH, which targets food and nutrients associated with lower risk of chronic disease).

The research team, led by Eric Rimm, ScD, associate professor of epidemiology and nutrition, and Stephanie Chiuve, ScD, research fellow in nutrition, prospectively monitored men in the Health Professionals Follow-up Study. The study documented 2,183 coronary events.

Researchers concluded that 62% of those coronary events may have been prevented if all men in the study population adhered to all five healthy lifestyle factors; for those men taking medications, 57% may have been prevented. Men who adopted two or more risk-lowering lifestyle factors during the study period had a 27% lower risk of CHD, compared to those making no changes. Overall, for each healthy lifestyle factor, the study found an inverse association with CHD risk.

The research is the first to look at the role of a healthy lifestyle and CHD in men in this age group. Chiuve says the study shows that "it's never too late to make changes to become healthier. You can still achieve benefits if you make changes in middle age or later in life."

To learn more: *Circulation*, July 11, 2006; abstract at <circ.ahajournals.org/cgi/content/abstract/114/2/160>. Alternate Healthy Eating Index <www.hsph.harvard.edu/nutritionsource/ pyramids.html>.

Shifting Carbs, Protein & Fats Cuts Heart Risk

The shifting scientific story on "carbs" in your diet took another twist at the American Heart Association's recent Scientific Sessions: Results from the OmniHeart study presented at the conference showed that substituting protein or monounsaturated fats for 10% of carbohydrates in an already healthy diet can reduce heart-disease risk. The findings suggest a possible improvement in the Dietary Approaches to Stop Hypertension (DASH) diet, which has been viewed as the "gold standard" in hypertension-fighting nutrition since the mid-1990s.

"Both the general public and the scientific research community are extremely interested in the health effects of shifting calories from carbohydrates," said Lawrence J. Appel, MD, professor of medicine at Johns Hopkins University and lead author of the study, which was published simultaneously in the *Journal of the American Medical Association.* "Our study provides evidence that substituting carbohydrates with protein (about half from plants) or with unsaturated fat (mostly monounsaturated fat) can lower blood pressure, improve cholesterol levels, and reduce heart disease risk."

Rather than studying the standard American diet, researchers tested three healthy diets. "All three diets are good; it's just that two of these diets are somewhat better," said Frank Sacks, MD, lead investigator from the study center at Brigham & Women's Hospital, Harvard Medical School. "These diets improved the whole cardiovascular risk spectrum. A lot of patients are tough to control with the medications we have. Patients might not even need drugs if they go on these diets."

Researchers studied 164 adults, average age 53.6, most of whom had elevated blood pressure not requiring medication ("prehypertension") and 21% of whom had hypertension. Just over half were African American, a population that has a greater-than-average risk of developing hypertension. Rather than comparing the reduced-carbohydrate diets to the standard American diet, the researchers tested against a diet very close to the DASH plan, which has proven to lower blood pressure; the 2,000-calorie DASH diet emphasizes fruits, vegetables and low-fat or fat-free dairy products. Subjects tried each of three diets for six weeks, with a "washout period" in-between:

• The DASH-like diet, with 58% of calories from carbohydrates, 15% from protein and 27% from fat (13% from monounsaturated fat).

• A diet shifting 10% of calories from carbs to protein, with 48% of calories from carbohydrates, 25% protein and 27% fat; about half of the protein came from plant sources such as beans, nuts and seeds and vegetable-based meat substitutes, plus roughly six ounces per day of chicken, fish, meat and egg-product-substitutes, all low in saturated fat.

• A diet shifting 10% of calories to unsaturated fat, mostly olive and canola oils, with 48% of calories from carbohydrates, 15% protein and 37% fat (21% monounsaturated fat).

All of the diets were extremely low in saturated fat (6% of calories). Researchers kept the patients' weight and exercise levels the same.

Compared to baseline levels, all three diets lowered systolic blood pressure by 8.2 mm Hg to 9.5 mm Hg and low-density lipoprotein (LDL) or "bad cholesterol" by 11.6 milligrams per deciliter (mg/dL). The protein diet further reduced systolic blood pressure by 1.4 mm Hg overall and lowered LDL by 3.3 mg/dL overall; it also significantly decreased high density lipoptotein (HDL)—the "good cholesterol"—however. The unsaturated-fat diet reduced systolic blood pressure by 1.3 mmHg more than the DASH diet; it had no significant effect on LDL but raised levels of HDL by 1.1 mg/dL. Both test diets reduced triglycerides (another fat in the blood), with the protein diet having a larger effect.

Researchers estimated each diet's effect on the 10-year risk of coronary heart disease based on well-established formulas. While all three diets lowered risk, the researchers concluded that the risk was lowest for people following the protein and the unsaturated-fat diets. Compared to baseline, each diet reduced heart disease risk—16% reduction in the DASH-like diet and about 20% reduction in the carb-cutting unsaturated fat and protein diets.

"There are many aspects of diet that we know affect heart disease risk," added Dr. Appel. "This study provides convincing evidence that the amount of carbohydrates, protein and fat people eat also influence risk."

To learn more: *Journal of the American Medical Association*, Nov. 16, 2005. Free abstract online at <jama.ama-assn.org/cgi/content/abstract/ 294/19/2455>. American Heart Association <www.americanheart.org/presenter.jhtml?identifier=3035497>.

"Five a Day" Reduces Risk of Stroke

Eating more than five portions of fruit and vegetables per day can cut the risk of stroke by 26%, according to new analysis published in *The Lancet*. Researchers examined data from eight studies (four from the US, three from Europe and one from Japan) that tracked the diets and occurrence of stroke among a total of 257,551 adults, followed for an average of 13 years. During that time, 4,917 of the subjects suffered a stroke.

People in the studies who regularly ate three to five servings a day of fruits and vegetables were 11% less likely to experience a stroke than those who ate fewer than three servings a day. And those whose diets routinely contained the most fruit and vegetables—more than five servings daily—were 26% less likely to suffer a stroke than those who ate the least.

The so-called "Five-A-Day" campaign to encourage eating more fruits and vegetables is well known, but recent studies have shown that the average consumption by people in developed countries is only three portions a day.

"These findings provide strong support for the recommendations encouraging the public to consume more than five servings of fruit and vegetables per day," wrote lead author Feng He from St. George's University of London. "Since raised blood pressure is the major cause of stroke, the blood-pressure-lowering effect of potassium could be one of the major mechanisms contributing to a reduced risk of stroke with an increased fruit and vegetable intake."

To learn more: *The Lancet*, Jan. 28, 2006. Free abstract at <www.thelancet.com/journals/ lancet/article/ PIIS0140673606680690/abstract>. Produce for Better Health Foundation <www.5aday.org>. American Stroke Association <www.strokeassociation.org>.

Vitamin Trials Fail to Prevent Second Heart Attack

Some 35% of Americans take B vitamins—folic acid, B12 and B6—many in doses higher than those in multivitamin supplements. Until now, scientists had high hopes that those vitamins could help prevent heart attacks and strokes by lowering blood levels of homocysteine. Previous studies had linked high levels of this amino acid to heart disease, and some researchers even likened homocysteine to cholesterol as a key risk factor. By lowering homocysteine levels, they reasoned, you could lower a patient's cardiovascular risk—much as statin drugs help by reducing unhealthy cholesterol.

Two new clinical trials, however, did not support that hope. Along with a similar study published in 2004, the research put B vitamins to the test in a total of nearly 13,000 patients at high risk for heart attack or stroke. Unlike earlier research that merely observed patient populations, all three recent studies tested the B vitamin-homocysteine theory by giving one group supplements while giving placebos to a control group.

Just as predicted, the B vitamins drove down subjects' homocysteine levels, in some cases by nearly a third. But the studies found little difference in the number of heart attacks between those taking the vitamins and those on placebos.

"The consistency among the results leads to the unequivocal conclusion that there is no clinical benefit of the use of folic acid and vitamin B12 (with or without the addition of vitamin B6) in patients with established vascular disease," wrote Joseph Loscalzo, MD, PhD, of Brigham and Women's Hospital in Boston in an editorial accompanying the two new studies, published in the *New England Journal of Medicine*.

Even the patron of the homocysteine theory, Kilmer McCully, MD, of the VA Boston Health Care System, agreed with that assessment. Dr. McCully first proposed a link between homocysteine levels and heart disease in 1969, an idea that slowly took hold over the next 25 years. But now, he told *The New York Times*, "The evidence is clear that this type of vitamin therapy is really not effective in reversing or benefiting advanced vascular disease."

Tufts experts, however, point out that these studies pertain only to those who already have heart disease.

The largest of the new studies, sponsored by the Canadian Institutes of Health Research, involved 5,522 patients age 55 or older with vascular disease or diabetes. They were randomly assigned to take either a placebo or a combination of 2.5 milligrams of folic acid, 50 milligrams of vitamin B6 and one milligram of B12, for an average of five years. The second new study, the Norwegian Vitamin Trial, involved 3,749 recent heart-attack victims, ages 30 to 85, over more than three years. In the 2004 Vitamin Intervention for Stroke Prevention trial, 3,680 stroke patients were tested for more than six years.

Though the vitamins showed some benefits, that was offset by increased risk of other health problems. The Norwegian researchers actually found a 22% increase—barely statistically significant—in risk of stroke, heart attack or heart-related death among subjects taking all three B vitamins.

So why does homocysteine seem to be associated with heart disease—but reducing blood levels by taking vitamin B doesn't help heart patients? Salim Yusuf, PhD, of McMaster University, a co-author of the Canadian study, speculated that scientists may have been confusing a symptom with a cause: Much as fever is a sign of infection, high homocysteine may be a red flag for heart disease—but not a cause of disease.

Older adults, whose bodies are not able to absorb vitamins B6 and B12 as effectively, may still need to supplement their intake from food.

To learn more: *New England Journal of Medicine,* April 13, 2006; online at <content. nejm.org> . *Journal of the American Medical Association,* Feb. 4, 2004; abstract online at <jama.ama-assn.org/ cgi/content/abstract/291/5/565>. NIH Office of Dietary Supplements Fact Sheets <dietary-supplements.info.nih.gov/ Health_ Information/ Information_About_Individual_Dietary_ Supplements.aspx>.

Heart Association Re-Assesses Data on Soy Protein's Benefits

In a turnaround that shouldn't come as a big surprise to readers of the *Healthletter*, the American Heart Association (AHA) has concluded that soy protein has little or no effect on risk factors for heart disease—though it can still be a healthful replacement for animal protein high in saturated fat. We previously spotlighted growing doubts about soy protein, once touted as a "magic bullet" against a variety of health problems. Now the AHA has officially joined those backing off from the soy bandwagon, updating a 2000 scientific statement that endorsed soy protein's potential for reducing cardiovascular risk.

The new statement, published in its journal *Circulation*, comes after an association committee analyzed data from 22 clinical trials. The analysis found that large amounts of soy protein in the diet reduced LDL ("bad") cholesterol only 3% and had no effect on HDL ("good") cholesterol, lipoprotein(a) or blood pressure. Additional analysis of 19 studies showed that soy isoflavones, the bioactive molecules found in soy, had no effect on LDL, triglycerides or HDL.

"A big LDL-lowering effect from soy protein or the isoflavones didn't happen," said Frank M. Sacks, MD, professor of nutrition at the Harvard School of Public Health in Boston. "In fact, the isoflavones did not lower LDL nor were there any proven positive biological effects in humans."

Among the experts preparing the update for the AHA's Nutrition Committee was Alice Lichtenstein, DSc, director of the Cardiovascular Nutrition Laboratory at Tufts' Jean Mayer USDA Human Nutrition Research Center on Aging.

The heart association committee also found that soy protein and isoflavones did not lessen menopause symptoms such as "hot flashes." The update added that evidence from clinical trials of soy isoflavones for the prevention or treatment of breast, endometrial and prostate cancer is "meager and cautionary," citing possible adverse effects. Results were mixed on claims that soy might slow postmenopausal bone loss.

"There are products in the market touting soy isoflavones and the phytoestrogens for issues related to women's health such as hot flashes, breast cancer and menopause," Dr. Sacks said. "There is nothing proven in this regard; there is little effect on hot flashes, and the osteoporosis prevention effects are mixed."

An earlier analysis of studies by the Agency for Healthcare Research and Quality (AHRQ)'s Tufts-New England Medical Center Evidence-Based Practice Center came to similar conclusions about soy protein's cholesterol-fighting effects. The majority of the soy isoflavone studies suggest that it might reduce the frequency of hot flashes in postmenopausal women, but Tufts' Joseph Lau, MD, co-author of the report, cautions, "the quality of the studies was poor and the long-term benefits remain unclear." The AHRQ analysis of 31 studies of soy and bone health failed to find sufficient data to suggest a benefit against postmenopausal bone loss.

Use of isoflavone supplements is not recommended, the AHA committee said, adding that earlier research indicateing soy protein had clinically favorable effects as compared to other proteins has not been confirmed.

Does this mean you should stop eating soy products? No—just don't expect miracles. The AHA statement still held out hope for benefits from soy-protein products such as tofu, soy butter, soy nuts and soy burgers. That's because soy protein can replace other high-fat proteins in the diet. "Soy products may have benefits when replacing other foods such as hamburgers," Dr. Sacks said. "Soy burgers have no cholesterol or saturated fat and have high amounts of fiber."

To learn more: American Heart Association
<www.americanheart.org/presenter.jhtml?identifier=3037031>.

Coffee Drinkers Perk Up Over Latest Findings
But decaf linked to higher cholesterol, colas to hypertension

If health concerns have caused you to switch to decaf coffee, new research may make you rethink your choices—especially if you're also swigging colas instead of regular java. One new study found that drinking decaffeinated coffee—but not caffeinated coffee—may be linked to higher levels of LDL, the "bad cholesterol." A second study exonerated coffee from a popularly held association with hypertension, at least for women, but identified a surprising connection between cola consumption and risk of high blood pressure.

The clear winner in this latest round of research, in short, is plain old caffeinated coffee—black, of course, hold the cream and sugar.

The first study, presented at the American Heart Association's Scientific Sessions, randomly assigned 187 people among three groups: one that drank three to six cups of caffeinated coffee daily; one that consumed the same amount of decaf; and a third that went coffee-free for three months.

Only the decaf group experienced a significant rise in two key factors associated with high LDL: ApoB, a protein attached to LDL and a predictor of cardiovascular disease risk, went up 8%, while non-esterified fatty acids (NEFA), fat in the blood that can fuel LDL production, rose an average of 18%. Neither ApoB nor NEFA significantly changed in the other two groups.

Lead author H. Robert Superko, MD, of the Fuqua Heart Center and the Piedmont-Mercer Center for Health and Learning in Atlanta, suspects that the difference in effects between decaf and regular coffee isn't the absence of caffeine. "Caffeinated and decaffeinated coffees are often made from different species of beans," he explains. "Caffeinated coffee, by and large, comes from a bean species called coffee Arabica, while many decaffeinated coffees are made from coffee Robusta. The decaffeination process can extract flavonoids and ingredients that give coffee flavor. So decaffeinated brands usually use a bean that has a more robust flavor."

If he's right, that also might be an argument for upgrading your coffee brand: Gourmet coffees are made from only Arabica beans, while cheaper supermarket brands use Robusta.

In any case, Dr. Superko says, "If you only drink one cup each day, the results of our study probably have little relevance."

To learn more: American Heart Association
<www.americanheart.org/presenter.jhtml?identifier=3035336>.
Journal of the American Medical Association, Nov. 9, 2005.
Free abstract at <jama. ama-assn.org/cgi/content/abstract/294/18/2330>.

Large Study Sees No Coffee-Heart Disease Connection

Go ahead, have another cup of coffee. A newly published study that followed some 120,000 men and women for up to 20 years has found no link between coffee consumption and higher risk of coronary heart disease (CHD).

The researchers, at Harvard University and the Universidad Autonoma in Madrid, did find that heavy coffee drinkers tend to have a lot of unhealthy habits. Java junkies were much more likely to smoke and drink alcohol, and less likely to exercise. But when those and other risk factors for heart disease were accounted for, simply drinking coffee—even lots of it—did not prove to be related to higher risk of CHD. The strong correlation with smoking, the investigators speculated, may explain why a previous study using data from the British National Health Service found a link between coffee drinking and heart disease, since smoking is a known risk factor for heart disease.

The new study, published in the American Heart Association journal *Circulation*, followed 44,005 men enrolled in the Health Professionals Follow-Up Study and 84,488 women in the Nurses' Health Study. Coffee consumption was first assessed in 1986 for men and in 1980 for women, and then every two to four years thereafter. A total of 2,173 cases of CHD were documented among the men and 2,254 among the women.

The research team cautioned, however, that their findings apply only to standard drip coffee. Earlier studies have "consistently shown that drinking a lot of French-press coffee increases LDL" (the "bad" cholesterol), according to co-author Rob van Dam, PhD, of the Harvard School of Public Health. It's also possible, he warned, that small groups of people with a particular genetic makeup might raise their CHD risk by drinking coffee.

To learn more: *Circulation*, May 2, 2006, abstract at
<circ.ahajournals.org/cgi/content/abstract/ 113/17/2045>.

Green Tea Brews
Cardiovascular Benefits

Have you had your green tea today? A large Japanese study of the effects of green-tea consumption on mortality suggests that several cups a day may help you have more tomorrows.

The study, published in the *Journal of the American Medical Association,* found that people who drank five or more cups of green tea daily had a 16% lower risk of death from all causes than those averaging less than one cup a day. (A cup in Japan is 3.3 ounces, not 6-8 as in the US.) The apparent benefits were more pronounced for death from cardiovascular disease—a 26% lower risk for the most avid green-tea drinkers—and seemed particularly effective against clot-related strokes.

Results for any possible cancer-fighting effect of green tea were disappointing, however, with no association between consumption and cancer mortality. No significant benefit for any type of mortality was seen from black or oolong tea.

"This report is, of course, constrained by the usual limitations of observational studies," cautions Jeffrey B. Blumberg, PhD, chief of the antioxidants research laboratory at Tufts' Jean Mayer USDA Human Nutrition Research Center on Aging. "However, the results are consistent with some

Green Tea and the "Asian Paradox"

Why don't people in Asian countries, where smoking is often even more common than in the US, suffer heart disease and lung cancer at the same high rates as Americans? One possible puzzle-piece to help explain this "Asian paradox," researchers at Yale University suggest, may be green tea. The antioxidants called catechins that are plentiful in Asian-preferred green tea, which is less processed than the black tea popular in the US, may have some protective effect. Writing in the *Journal of the American College of Surgeons*, Bauer E. Sumpio, MD, PhD, and colleagues say the antioxidants may help keep artery walls functioning properly, inhibit clots and even block tumor growth or formation.

To highlight the "Asian paradox," the researchers point to Japan and Korea. In Japan, which has a higher rate of smoking than the US, the annual death rate from coronary heart disease per 100,000 men is 186, compared to 348 in the US. The rate of lung cancer deaths among Korean women is 13 per 100,000; among Korean men, 40 per 100,000. That compares to 45 and 67 per 100,000, respectively, for US women and men—even though 37% of Koreans smoke, versus 27% of Americans.

Don't take the possible benefits of green tea as a green light to smoke, however. Not every comparison shows the "Asian paradox": China has a higher coronary death rate than the US, and Japanese and American men are about equally prone to die of lung cancer. Says Dr. Sumpio, "Smoking cessation is the best way to prevent cardiovascular disease and cancer."

To learn more: *Journal of the American College of Surgeons*, May 2006.

animal model and small clinical studies and that makes the story a bit more compelling." In prior studies, the strongest scientific evidence for benefits from tea consumption has been for reducing heart disease. Blumberg says, "Heavy tea drinkers have a lower risk of heart disease—the data are very consistent."

The new Japanese research, a population-based prospective study begun in 1994, followed 40,530 adults ages 40 to 79 in northeastern Japan. Over 11 years of follow-up, 4,209 subjects died from all causes; during a seven-year period, 892 died of cardiovascular disease and 1,134 of cancer. Small apparent benefits from green-tea consumption were found with as little as one to two cups a day (5% reduced all-cause mortality compared to those drinking the least).

The link between green tea and reduced mortality was strongest among women. Researchers speculated that the gender gap may be due in part to cigarette smoking, still common among men in Japan. Because green-tea consumption is so prevalent in Japan—80% of the population in the study area drink green tea—researchers said it was unlikely that the results were otherwise skewed by healthier lifestyles among green-tea drinkers.

The exact mechanism of green tea's health benefits is unknown, but researchers suggested it may be related to the high levels of polyphenols—natural antioxidants—in green tea.

To learn more: Journal of the American Medical Association, Sept. 13, 2006; abstract at <jama.ama-assn.org/cgi/content/abstract/296/10/1255>.

Chocolate Bars Promise Heart-Health Bonus

Can a candy bar be good for you? Mars Inc., the maker of M&Ms and Snickers, certainly thinks so. In 2003, the company created the CocoaVia snack bar, which it promotes as packed with cocoa flavanols—antioxidants that may have heart-healthy qualities. Now it's also introduced a variety of new CocoaVia chocolate bars and rolled out retail sales nationwide; originally, the bars—priced at about $1 each—were available only online.

"CocoaVia is the vanguard of our efforts to 'reinvent' cocoa as an ingredient in healthful foods," says Harold Schmitz, PhD, chief science officer at Mars. "It's a first-of-its-kind product that was purposely designed to deliver heart-health benefits and real chocolate pleasure in products that are less than 150 calories per serving."

Each CocoaVia bar—the company recommends eating two daily—contains 100 milligrams of cocoa flavanols plus 1.1 grams of canola sterol esters. According to the US Food and Drug Administration, a daily total intake of at least 1.3 grams of such phytosterols, as part of a diet low in saturated fat and cholesterol, may reduce the risk of heart disease.

But nutrition experts point out that these healthful ingredients come at a price—in calories and saturated fat. A CocoaVia bar contains a relatively modest 100 calories (140 in a serving of the new CocoaVia-covered almonds), about which Mars carefully notes, "Since each serving is packed with the heart-healthy flavanols, you can eat a relatively small portion and still reap the benefits. That means less fat and fewer calories compared to a regular, larger-sized chocolate bar." In blunter terms, you're getting a 0.78-ounce chocolate bar that's barely over half the size of a regular, 1.5-ounce Hershey bar. Ounce for ounce, CocoaVia has 84% of the calories in chocolate candy.

Whatever CocoaVia's cholesterol-lowering benefits, keep in mind that each bar also contains 3.5 grams of saturated fat (per ounce, three-quarters the amount in ordinary chocolate). In a two-bar daily dose, that's 36% of the daily value of this key contributor to unhealthy blood cholesterol.

To learn more: CocoaVia <www.cocoavia.com>.

Pendulum Swings on Estrogen and Women's Heart Health Risk

New research into the benefits and risks of Hormone Replacement Therapy (HRT) may allow women entering menopause to reconsider their options. Findings recently published in the *Journal of Women's Health* show that women who began HRT soon after entering menopause had a 30% lower risk for heart disease than women who did not use hormones. Contrary to earlier research linking estrogen treatment to increased cardiovascular risks, this Harvard analysis of data from the Nurses Health Study indicates HRT may indeed offer heart-protective benefits, depending on a woman's age and how long since she entered menopause.

Publication of this research was swiftly followed by a fresh analysis of

Hormone Replacement Therapy: What Should You Do?

Latest advice from the Women's Health Initiative for menopausal women:

• Discuss these findings with your doctor in regard to your own health.

• Do not take hormone therapy to prevent heart disease. Instead, talk with your doctor about other ways to protect your heart. If you take hormone therapy to help prevent osteoporosis, ask your doctor about other ways to help preserve bone and slow down bone loss.

• If you decide to use hormones, use them at the lowest dose that helps and for the shortest time needed. Check with your doctor every three to six months to see if you still need them.

the Women's Health Initiative (WHI) data that first raised concerns about HRT in 2002. This updated analysis, published in the *Archives of Internal Medicine,* suggests that health concerns about menopause hormones may have been overstated. WHI project officer Jacques Rossouw said the findings should reassure women who might be weighing the risks against the benefits of HRT for menopause symptoms.

The latest WHI analysis focused on 10,739 women in the nearly seven-year study who used only estrogen. Overall, it found neither added cardiovascular risks nor benefits from estrogen use. But the youngest women studied, ages 50 to 59, did have a 45% reduced risk of angioplasty or bypass surgery.

That contrasts sharply with the original findings in the government-funded HRT study, which was halted in 2002 prior to completion when an independent safety board observed a significant incidence of cardiovascular events, deep-vein thrombosis, pulmonary embolism and heart disease. The board concluded the risks of taking HRT outweighed the possible benefits. That news widely swayed the thinking of women and their doctors, and sales of estrogen drugs—at that time the second most widely prescribed drug in the US—plunged by half.

Since then, however, a number of researchers have questioned that alarm. For one thing, the design of the study didn't necessarily apply to typical hormone users—women who turn to the drugs to relieve standard menopausal symptoms, including night sweats, insomnia and vaginal dryness. In fact, most women in the study were more than 10 years past menopause.

Both new publications suggest that age may be a factor in the estrogen-cardiovascular equation. The Harvard researchers found no heart benefit for older nurses who began HRT 10 or more years after menopause. Likewise, while the youngest women in the updated WHI analysis were less likely to need cardiovascular surgeries, those who began HRT past age 60 showed no heart benefits; women age 70-plus appeared to suffer increased heart risks, much like the older women in the original 2002 findings.

Neither of the new reports indicates a woman should take HRT solely to lower her risk of heart attack. They do suggest, however, that women suffering from hot flashes and other symptoms of menopause shouldn't fear increased risk of heart disease if they decide to use hormones for relief.

But Harvard epidemiologist Francine Grodstein, DSc, lead author of the *Journal of Women's Health* study, cautions against jumping back on the estrogen bandwagon. She says the findings "should not change anyone's mind regarding medical practice," and that the "statistics should only serve to generate more research."

That's exactly what's happening, in fact: The Kronos Longevity Research Institute has launched the Kronos Early Estrogen Prevention Study (KEEPS) to examine whether starting hormone therapy in early menopause helps protect women from heart disease. WHI researchers are also expected to publish a further analysis of younger women in the study who began HRT shortly after entering menopause.

To learn more: *Journal of Women's Health,* January 2006; free article online at
<www.liebertonline. com/doi/pdf/10.1089/jwh.2006.15.35>.
Archives of Internal Medicine, Feb. 13, 2006; free abstract online at
<archinte.ama-assn.org/cgi/content/abstract/ 166/3/357>. Women's Health Initiative
<www. 4woman.gov/menopause/news.htm>. KEEPS <www.kronosinstitute.org/keeps.html>.

Q Frankly, I'm getting real tired of being told I don't know what I'm talking about. My husband and I both have high cholesterol. My husband is a hunter, and he and his buddies claim that wild meat is good and OK to eat as much as one wants. I say red meat is red meat regardless. If I'm wrong, fine, I'll accept it; if not, then they will be stuck with more chicken, fish or turkey dishes.

A We suggest your husband should spend some time fishing as well as hunting. Just because meat is wild rather than farm-raised doesn't magically make it good for you; moderation is still the key to healthy eating. All meat contains some fat, saturated fat and cholesterol—plus of course calories.

That being said, however, it's true that game meats in general are leaner than many cuts of red meat you might buy at the grocery store. For example, according to the USDA's Nutrient Data Laboratory <www.ars.usda.gov/ba/bhnrc/ndl>, a three-ounce serving of venison steak contains just 128 calories, 2 grams total fat, 0.8 gram of saturated fat and 67 milligrams of cholesterol. Compare that to the same size portion of beef porterhouse steak—202 calories, almost 15 grams total fat, a whopping 6.8 grams saturated fat and 54 milligrams of cholesterol.

You'll note that venison, like most game meats, is relatively higher in cholesterol. Organ meats, whether wild or domestic, are also extremely high in cholesterol. While this is something to watch, cholesterol in food is not the only contributor to your LDL ("bad") cholesterol blood levels. According to the American Heart Association, dietary saturated fat is the main culprit in LDL cholesterol; game meats in general are lower in saturated fat than comparable cuts of beef or pork.

Among the leaner varieties of wild game red meat are deer, elk, antelope, wild boar, squirrel and rabbit; bear meat is relatively high in fat. Choose carefully among wild birds, however: Pheasant, quail, wild turkey and dove are all similar to or slightly leaner than chicken, but duck and goose (wild or domestic) are much higher in cholesterol and saturated fat.

If your husband went fishing for rainbow trout instead, a three-ounce serving would contain only 101 calories, 0.6 gram of saturated fat and 50 milligrams of cholesterol.

The Lowdown on
High Blood Pressure

Shaking the Salt Habit

Reducing the sodium in your diet can lower your risk of high blood pressure and other serious ailments.

You pass on using the shaker at the table and use a variety of herbs and spices in place of salt when you cook. Can you still be getting too much of the white stuff?

Absolutely. The federal government's National High Blood Pressure Education Program (NHBPEP) recommends that adults consume no more than 2,400 milligrams of sodium per day, which is about the amount in a teaspoon of salt. The government Dietary Guidelines for Americans updated in 2005 are even stricter, saying people should consume fewer than 2,300 milligrams daily, and that those with high blood pressure, African-Americans and middle-aged and older adults should get only two-thirds of that amount of sodium. The American Heart Association (AHA) advises people with heart disease to consume no more than 2,000 milligrams of sodium per day.

These are broad-brush recommendations. Individuals respond differently to sodium, and you may be more or less sensitive to its effects than average. In general, though, less sodium is better for your health.

How much better? A recent report by Britain's Medical Research Council (MRC) estimates that a 37% reduction in that nation's sodium consumption—which is even higher than in the US—would result in a 13% reduction in stroke and a 10% decrease in the incidence of heart disease.

Research recently presented at the American Heart Association's Scientific Sessions shows specifically how cutting back on dietary salt intake can reduce the risk of heart disease. Back in 1987 to 1995, as part of a nationwide trial, men and women ages 30 to 54 with high normal blood pressure learned how to identify, select and prepare low-salt foods. Researchers at Brigham and

Kitchen Chemistry Lesson

You'll often hear the terms "salt" and "sodium" used interchangeably, but they're not exactly the same thing. Chemically speaking, salt consists of 40% sodium and 60% chlorine. Remember the NaCl formula from your high school chemistry class? The "Na" (from the Latin "natrium") stands for sodium, the "Cl" for chlorine. Even though it takes one of each to make a salt molecule, the atomic weight of chlorine is roughly half again as much as that of sodium, so chlorine makes up 60% of the weight of salt.

That means that if you want to convert an amount of salt to sodium, you need to divide the salt figure by 2.5; to convert sodium to salt, multiply by 2.5. So 1,000 milligrams of salt would be 400 milligrams of sodium; 1,000 milligrams of sodium would be 2,500 milligrams of salt. The amount of sodium that the government dietary guidelines recommend as the maximum per day–2,300 milligrams–would be contained in 5,750 milligrams of salt, about one teaspoon.

Women's Hospital in Boston followed up with the participants and found that those who reduced their sodium intake had lowered their subsequent risk of cardiovascular disease or death by 26%. The researchers also found that a higher average intake of sodium was associated with increased risk of later cardiovascular events.

"A decrease in sodium in the diet, even among those with only modestly elevated blood pressure, lowers risk of cardiovascular disease later in life," says Brigham and Women's researcher Nancy Cook, DSc.

Hypertension and Other Risks

The primary threat from too much salt in your diet is high blood pressure, which is a major risk factor for cardiovascular disease—the nation's number-one killer. Salt increases blood pressure because its sodium—one of salt's two "ingredients" (for the difference between salt and sodium, see the box below)—makes the body retain extra water. The additional water in the blood vessels creates more pressure. To pump the added fluid, the heart has to work harder, putting an added strain on your heart.

About 65 million people have high blood pressure, according to a recent study published in the journal *Circulation*. Those with normal blood pressure at age 55 nonetheless have a 90% chance of eventually developing hypertension, defined as a blood-pressure reading of 140/90 or higher.

According to Stephen Havas, MD, MPH, MS, vice president for science, quality and public health for the American Medical Association, 700,000 Americans die each year of heart disease and more than 160,000 die of stroke. "Those who don't consume a healthy diet are putting their lives at risk," says Dr. Havas, who also represents the American Public Health Association on an expert committee that advises the National Institutes of

Health on hypertension.

He adds that an estimated 150,000 lives are lost each year directly attributable to excess sodium consumption. "Unfortunately, a lifetime of eating too much salt is needlessly increasing the risk of dying from cardio-vascular disease." Sodium consumption, Dr. Havas says, is "the driving force" behind hypertension in particular.

Where the Salt Is–and Isn't

Only a small amount of sodium occurs naturally in foods; most of the sodium in your diet gets added in processing. This table from the DASH Eating Plan gives examples of the amounts of sodium in some foods:

Food Groups	Sodium (milligrams)
Grains and Grain Products	
Cooked cereal, rice, pasta, unsalted, 1/2 cup	0-5
Ready-to-eat cereal, 1 cup	100-360
Bread, 1 slice	110-175
Vegetables	
Fresh or frozen, cooked without salt, 1/2 cup	1-70
Canned or frozen with sauce, 1/2 cup	140-460
Tomato juice, canned, 3/4 cup	820
Fruit	
Fresh, frozen, canned, 1/2 cup	0-5
Lowfat or Fat-Free Dairy Foods	
Milk, 1 cup	120
Yogurt, 8 ounces	160
Natural cheeses, 1 1/2 ounces	110-450
Processed cheeses, 1 1/2 ounces	600
Nuts, Seeds, and Dry Beans	
Peanuts, salted, 1/3 cup	120
Peanuts, unsalted, 1/3 cup	0-5
Beans, cooked from dried, or frozen, without salt, 1/2 cup	0-5
Beans, canned, 1/2 cup	400
Meats, Fish, and Poultry	
Fresh meat, fish, poultry, 3 ounces	30-90
Tuna canned, water pack, no salt added, 3 ounces	35-45
Tuna canned, water pack, 3 ounces	250-350
Ham, lean, roasted, 3 ounces	1,020

Besides a heart attack, hypertension also increases your risk of stroke and kidney disease. Too much salt can worsen symptoms such as swelling and shortness of breath and cause weight gain. Extremely high salt con-sumption affects bone health and may contribute to stomach cancer.

Pregnant women have also long been cautioned to cut back on salt to avoid preeclampsia, a toxic condition associated with swelling and elevated blood pressure, usually late in a pregnancy. More recent studies, however, have found that sodium consumption close to or below the adequate intake of 1.5 grams per day seems to have no effect on whether preeclampsia occurs. "Thus, the recommended intake for sodium during pregnancy is the

Potent Potassium

Potassium just might be the anti-salt, it turns out. "Diets rich in potassium not only reduce blood pressure, but also blunt some of the rise in blood pressure that occurs in response to sodium intake," according to Lawrence Appel, MD, MPH, professor of medicine, epidemiology and international health at Johns Hopkins Medical Institutions. "High intakes of potassium also reduce bone loss and can prevent kidney stone recurrence in men and women." Potassium also helps to reduce irregular heart beats suffered by those with congestive heart failure.

The National Academies' Dietary Reference Intakes for Water, Potassium, Sodium, Chloride and Sulfate, a report developed by American and Canadian scientists and released in 2004, as well as the Dietary Guidelines for Americans 2005, recommend that people consume 4,700 milligrams of potassium each day from fruits, vegetables and juices. No upper limit was set. That's a lot of potassium: a cup of baked acorn squash, one of the richest potassium sources, has about 900 milligrams, while a banana has between 400 and 500 milligrams. Other fruits and vegetables to consider as potassium sources include spinach and other dark, leafy greens; cantaloupes; oranges; tomatoes; winter squash; potatoes; and beans. Almonds and dairy products are also good sources.

Remember in selecting your potassium sources to balance other concerns, such as sugar. And the Dietary References Intakes report noted that people with known kidney problems and on certain medications, such as those for high blood pressure, have to carefully monitor their potassium intake and should follow their health care professionals' advice rather than the general recommendations.

same as for nonpregnant women," the National Academies (which includes the National Academy of Science) said in its Dietary Reference Intakes for Water, Potassium, Sodium, Chloride and Sulfate in 2004.

Although sodium is an essential nutrient your body needs, Dr. Havas says no one fails to get enough from natural sources. In fact, the National Academies' Dietary Reference Intakes report in 2004 estimated that the Yanomamo Indians of Brazil survive with less than 200 milligrams per day of sodium. At the opposite extreme, the report noted that the average daily sodium intake in northern Japan is more than 10,300 milligrams per person—three times the average US level. (The Japanese diet also is typically heavy in potassium; for more on the yin and yang of potassium and sodium, see box above.)

How Much Is Too Much?

The US Food and Drug Administration (FDA) amended pending rules so that meals and main-dish products can call themselves "healthy" if they have 600 milligrams or less of sodium (480 milligrams for individual products); more restrictive levels had been scheduled to take effect. The FDA cited technological barriers to reducing sodium in processed foods and poor sales of products that did meet the proposed lower levels. In light of the government's own guideline of 2,300 milligrams of sodium daily, however, some health advocates say those higher levels don't exactly seem like an all-out war on salt.

That's what the British government has recently launched, following the MRC's findings about the health benefits there of slashing sodium intake. According to the MRC, the average Brit consumes a whopping 9,500 milligrams of salt per day (that's 3,800 milligrams of sodium). The national goal is to cut that amount to 6,000 milligrams of salt per day (or 2,400 milligrams of sodium) by 2010 for adults.

Salty Language

What's the difference between, say, "low sodium" and "reduced sodium"? Here's a quick rundown on the Food and Drug Administration's definitions of various sodium content terms:

Sodium free or salt free: Less than 5 milligrams (mg) per serving

Very low sodium: 35 mg or less of sodium per serving

Low sodium: 140 mg or less of sodium per serving

Reduced or less sodium: At least 25% less sodium than the regular version

Light in sodium: 50% less sodium than the regular version

Lightly salted: At least 50% less sodium per serving than reference amount

Unsalted, without added salt, no salt added: No salt added during processing, and the food it resembles and for which it substitutes is normally processed with salt

That's an ambitious goal. The MRC says a survey conducted in 2000-01 found that just 15% of British men and 31% of women consumed less than 2,400 milligrams of salt per day. And salt consumption has actually been rising in Britain: That 9,500 milligrams average was up from a 1986-7 study in which adults were taking in 9,000 milligrams of salt each day.

The government recently launched a public-awareness campaign that includes a television ad in which chicken curry, spaghetti sauce and other

Hunting Hidden Sodium

Britain's Medical Research Council suggests you watch out for these sodium-based food additives:

Additive	Use
Sodium citrate:	Flavoring, preservative
Sodium chloride:	Flavoring, texture, preservative
Monosodium glutamate:	Flavor enhancer
Sodium cyclamate:	Artificial sweetener
Sodium bicarbonate:	Yeast substitute
Sodium nitrate:	Preservative, color fixative

prepared foods vie for a shopper's attention. She makes her selection based on the salt content listed on the label. "Eat no more than six grams [6,000 milligrams] of salt a day," ends the ad from the Food Standards Agency, an independent department similar to the United States' FDA.

"Bringing our salt intake down to below the recommended level of six grams per day for adults will result in many thousands of lives saved in years to come," says Graham MacGregor, MD, professor of cardiovascular medicine at London's St. George's Hospital and chairman of England's Consensus Action on Salt and Health (CASH), a group of specialists concerned with salt and its effects on health.

Americans may not consume quite as much salt as the British, but most of us also have a way to go to reach our own government's guideline of no more than 2,300 milligrams of sodium daily. According to the recently released report, "What We Eat in America," based on data from the ongoing National Health and Nutrition Examination Survey (NHANES) compiled in 2001-02, the average American consumes 3,292 milligrams of sodium daily. The figures are worse for certain segments of the population: Males ages 31-50 consume the most sodium, a whopping 4,252 milligrams daily. Only infants, on average, are getting less than the recommended maximum of 2,300 milligrams a day. Overall, across all gender and age groups, 86% of Americans are consuming too much sodium, according to the report.

Richard L. Hanneman, president of the industry-sponsored Salt Institute, maintains that no medical studies have concluded that the health of people who consume salt at the rate we do in the US is at risk. He says sodium should be judged on its overall effects on health, not just blood pressure. He says it's plausible—though untested—that since salt intakes are relatively predictable and unchanging over time, "the body may use salt as a feed-limiter, turning on or off humans' appetite mechanism and affecting total food intake. If that would prove true, substituting low-sodium foods into the diet might not reduce total sodium, but might lead to increased caloric intake and contribute to overeating."

But Dr. Havas says the salt-calorie equation is exactly the other way around. Salt makes you thirsty, which causes you to drink more high-calorie fluids such as sodas and alcoholic beverages. "Why else do you think bars put out bowls of salty peanuts?"

How to Cut Back

In any case, most medical experts agree that reducing your sodium intake is an important step to better health. The only real question is how to do it?

The tricky part about shaking the salt habit is that as much as 90% of the salt you consume every day is "hidden"—salt that you don't shake on at the stovetop or the dining table. According to one tally, about 77% of the sodium in the average American diet comes from processed foods and restaurant foods. About 12% occurs naturally in foods such as dairy and seafood. Only 5% is added during cooking, and just 6% gets added at the table from your salt shaker.

For example, one cup of canned ham and bean soup comes in at 972 milligrams of sodium per serving. One company's individual-sized pan pizza has 983 milligrams of sodium per serving. One hamburger chain's signature burger has 1,070 milligrams, representing nearly half the upper limit of your recommended sodium for the day before you've even asked for fries (more salt, plus of course saturated fat and calories) or had something to drink. (That diet soda can add another 50 milligrams of sodium.)

If you're in the habit of eating on the run, whether it's via fast-food restaurants or heat-and-serve products at home, don't try to change your salt intake overnight. Salt adds flavor to food, and going to the opposite extreme cold turkey is a recipe for failure. As the FDA noted in amending its rules on sodium content in "healthy" food labels, some foods that are good for us aren't good for the manufacturers' bottom line. In another acknowledgement of that fact, the National Academies' Dietary Reference Intakes recommended additional research to guide the food industry in developing technologies that reduce prepared and processed foods' sodium content while maintaining food quality, acceptability and cost.

For success in cutting down on sodium, take a leaf from HHS's Dietary Approaches to Stop Hypertension, or DASH, Eating Plan. DASH is an outgrowth of research sponsored by the National Heart, Lung and Blood Institute (NHLBI). The plan, which is low in sodium, saturated fat, cholesterol and total fat, and emphasizes fruits, vegetables and low-fat dairy foods, is considered the best dietary blueprint against hypertension.

But even expert sources such as DASH and the American Heart Association recommend gradual change to retrain your tastebuds. For example, you might simply remove the salt shaker from your table or refrain from using the salt packet that came in the bag with your fast food. Rather than cutting out popcorn (which is a good source of whole grain), consider the brands that don't add salt or butter—or pop it yourself from kernels.

You can lose a lot of dietary sodium painlessly just by switching from canned vegetables to fresh or frozen produce. If you can't find affordable produce options, seek out reduced-sodium varieties of canned vegetables, as well as low-sodium chicken broth, soup and other packaged foods.

You can also cut the sodium in canned vegetables by draining and giving them a quick rinse: According to Steve Harrison at Bush Brothers, a packager of beans, for instance, the nutrition facts on a can of variety beans (chicken peas, kidney beans, etc.) assume the entire contents, the beans plus the brine. By simply draining the beans, you reduce the sodium content by approximately 40%, Harrison says, based on an analysis by an independent lab. A 30-second rinse with plain water reduces the sodium by about another 3%. In a simple can of beans, this two-step trick can reduce the sodium content per serving from a typical 400 milligrams to 228 milligrams.

As this example shows, it's important to read those nutrition labels! Unlike fat and fiber listings that can sometimes be confusing, sodium is a label line that's easy (albeit sometimes shocking) to read and understand. Just make sure you're aware of the serving size that goes with that sodium figure.

But the battle against sodium doesn't end at the supermarket. Many restaurant meals contain more than an entire day's worth of sodium. "Ask for low-salt alternatives when you order," suggests Dr. Havas. "And if they can't comply, switch restaurants."

Try these other sodium-cutting tips that we've culled from the DASH Eating Plan and the British Food Standards Agency:

• Use fresh poultry, fish and lean meat, rather than canned, smoked or processed types.

• Choose ready-to-eat breakfast cereals that are lower in sodium.

• Limit cured foods (such as bacon and ham), foods packed in brine (such as pickles, pickled vegetables, olives and sauerkraut) and condiments such as MSG, mustard, horseradish, catsup and barbecue sauce.

• Limit even lower-sodium versions of soy sauce and teriyaki sauce.

• Flavor foods with herbs, spices, lemon, lime, vinegar or salt-free seasoning blends.

• Cook rice, pasta and hot cereals without salt.

• Cut back on instant or flavored rice, pasta and cereal mixes, which usually have added salt.

• Cut back on frozen dinners, mixed dishes such as pizza, packaged mixes, canned soups or broths, and salad dressings—these often have a lot of sodium.

• Rinse canned foods such as tuna, to remove some sodium.

• Marinate meat and fish in advance to give them more flavor without salt.

- Add red wine to stews and casseroles, and white wine to risottos and sauces for chicken. (Don't make the mistake, however, of buying "cooking wine," which contains salt to make it undrinkable.)
- Make your own stock and gravy instead of using cubes or granules.

A DASH of Healthy Eating

Once you've had success with those modifications, you may wish to delve more deeply into a low-sodium lifestyle, such as that outlined in the DASH Eating Plan.

The research behind DASH was conducted at Brigham and Women's; Duke University Medical Center in Durham, NC; Johns Hopkins; and the Pennington Biomedical Research Center at Louisiana State University in Baton Rouge, beginning in 1994. It initially involved 459 adults with blood pressure below 160/80-95. Twenty percent had high blood pressure, about half were women, and 60% were African-American. Participants followed one of three eating plans—a typical diet; a typical diet higher in fruits and vegetables; and DASH—all of which had about 3,000 milligrams of sodium per day. Both DASH and the plan higher in fruits and vegetables reduced blood pressure, with DASH having the greater effect, particularly among those with high blood pressure.

In the next phase, from 1997 to 1999, 412 participants with blood pressure readings of 120-159/80-95 followed either DASH or a typical diet at one of three sodium levels (3,300, 2,400 and 1,500). "Results showed that reducing dietary sodium lowered blood pressure for both eating plans," the NHLBI says. "At each sodium level, blood pressure was lower on the DASH eating plan than on the other eating plan. The biggest blood pressure reductions were for the DASH eating plan at the sodium intake of 1,500 milligrams per day. Those with hypertension saw the biggest reductions, but those without it also had large decreases."

In an added benefit, "Those on the 1,500-milligram sodium intake eating plan, as well as those on the DASH eating plan, had fewer headaches," NHLBI says.

Recent research has found that modifying a DASH-like diet by switching 10% of calories from carbohydrates to protein or monounsaturated fat may make this healthy eating plan even better.

Remember that cutting back on salt is only part of the answer to fighting hypertension and its related health problems. You'll want to limit overall calories and maintain a healthy weight. It's important to also develop an exercise plan that fits your interests and your needs. And, just for fun, throw a pinch of that salt you're not using over your shoulder for luck!

To Learn More: Dietary Approaches to Stop Hypertension Eating Plan
<www.nhlbi.nih.gov/health/public/heart/hbp/dash>.

British 6-gram effort <www.salt.gov.uk> and <www.mrc.ac.uk>.
National Academies' Dietary Reference Intakes report and other scientific information of interest
<www.nationalacademies.org>. USDA Nutrient Data Laboratory <www.ars.usda.gov/ba/bhnrc/ndl>.
National High Blood Pressure Education Program <www.nhlbi. nih.gov/about/nhbpep>.
American Heart Association <www.americanheart.org/presenter.jhtml?identifier=2106> and
<www.americanheart.org/presenter. jhtml?identifier=336>.

Battling Poor Cholesterol Levels May Also Fight Hypertension

Here's yet another reason to control your cholesterol: Harvard researchers have linked high levels of total cholesterol to an increased risk of developing high blood pressure. The research also found an association between high HDL ("good" cholesterol) levels and significantly lower risk for hypertension.

"Our findings suggest we may have a new means of preventing hypertension, a devastating public health issue in this country," researcher Howard D. Sesso, DSc, MPH, an associate epidemiologist at Harvard Medical School and Brigham and Women's Hospital, told Reuters news service.

The study, published in *Hypertension*, looked at data on 3,110 men from the long-running Physicians' Health Study. About a third of the men, 1,019, developed hypertension over an average follow-up time of 14 years.

Although the latest study focused only on men, another recent study of 16,130 women, published in *Archives of Internal Medicine*, found similar results.

The researchers discovered that the men with the highest total cholesterol had a 23% greater risk of developing hypertension later in life than those with the lowest levels. Those with highest ratio of total cholesterol to HDL cholesterol were 54% more likely to later suffer high blood pressure.

Lead author Ruben O. Halperin, MD, MPH, wrote that poor cholesterol levels "appear to predate the onset of hypertension by years."

On the other hand, men with the highest levels of "good" HDL cholesterol had a 32% lower risk of developing hypertension than the group with the lowest HDL.

Dr. Halperin believes that measuring cholesterol levels in men could help determine whether they might be at risk for developing hypertension. The study "lends support to the theory that hypertension represents an early manifestation of the atherosclerotic process," he added. It may even be that controlling cholesterol by means of diet and medication such as statins could have an added benefit in helping to keep blood pressure from reaching dangerous levels.

To learn more: *Hypertension*, January 2006; free abstract at <hyper.ahajournals.org/cgi/content/abstract/47/1/45>. *Archives of Internal Medicine*, Nov. 14, 2005; free abstract at <archinte.ama-assn.org/cgi/content/ abstract/165/20/2420>. American Heart Association <www.americanheart.org/ presenter.jhtml?identifier=2114>.

Potassium Salt Substitute Found to Lower Heart Risk

There may be good news coming from an unexpected source—your salt shaker. A new report published in the *American Journal of Clinical Nutrition* suggests that replacing regular salt with a potassium-fortified alternative may help lower adults' risk of death from cardiovascular disease.

Nearly 2,000 elderly Taiwanese men in a veterans' retirement home were involved in the study. Nearly half were randomly assigned to eat meals prepared with potassium-enriched salt, while the others got food prepared with regular salt (sodium chloride). The researchers found that over the next 30 months, men given the salt alternative were 40% less likely to die from cardiovascular disease.

The salt alternative, composed of half sodium chloride and half potassium chloride, enabled the men to moderately cut their sodium intake while simultaneously boosting their potassium intake. The beneficial effects of a lower sodium diet have been well documented. But it was likely the increased potassium—a nutrient thought to offer protection to blood-vessel function—that lowered the risk of cardiovascular death, according to study co-author Wen-Harn Pan, PhD, a researcher at the Institute of Biomedical Sciences, Academia Sinica, in Taipei, Taiwan.

Potassium is an electrolyte, like sodium, necessary for maintaining the body's fluid balance. Involved in proper nerve function and muscle control, potassium also helps regulate blood pressure.

While the study looked at potassium-enriched salt, Pan told Reuters Health that she believes a diet high in potassium-rich fruits and vegetables could be even more beneficial; whole foods contain other nutrients important to overall health. Potassium-enriched salt offers a "convenient and fast way" to alter the diet's sodium-potassium ratio, however.

The Morton salt company and others make low-sodium table salt, a sodium chloride and potassium chloride mix. The commercially available product contains 50% less sodium than regular salt.

A word of caution, though: It is possible to overdose on potassium. Particularly at risk are older people with kidney dysfunction or who are taking ACE inhibitors for their blood pressure. Check with your doctor before using potassium-enriched salt substitutes.

To learn more: *American Journal of Clinical Nutrition,* June 2006; abstract at
<www.ajcn.org/cgi/content/abstract/83/6/1289>.

Coffee Cleared in Hypertension–
But What About Cola?

Coffee drinkers can perk up at the results of an analysis of hypertension and caffeine intake in 155,594 women in the two Nurses Health Studies (NHS). The study, published in the *Journal of the American Medical Association,* aimed in part to test the popular assumption that drinking coffee can lead to high blood pressure.

The researchers found "no distinct and positive association" between coffee and hypertension. In fact, they identified a slight possible protective effect: Women who drank the most coffee—more than six cups a day—showed a 9-12% lesser risk of hypertension than those averaging less than a cup a day.

No similar large study has been conducted on men, although a 2002 study of 1,017 men linked coffee to small increases in blood pressure but not to the development of hypertension.

This new NHS analysis also looked at tea consumption, with no conclusive results, and at cola consumption. That's where scientists got a surprise.

Lead author Wolfgang Winkelmayer, MD, ScD, of Brigham and Women's Hospital in Boston, says, "We found a very consistent, direct and positive association between cola drinks and the risk of hypertension." Women consuming more than four cans daily of sugared cola showed an increased risk of 28-44% compared to those drinking less than one can a day. The group that drank the most sugar-free cola had a 16-19% greater hypertension risk.

Until a biological mechanism is uncovered to explain the cola-hypertension connection, Dr. Winkelmayer said, it's premature to suggest women change their beverage choices.

To learn more: American Heart Association
<www.americanheart.org/presenter.jhtml?identifier=3035336>.
Journal of the American Medical Association, Nov. 9, 2005. Free abstract at
<jama. ama-assn.org/cgi/content/abstract/294/18/2330>.

Low-Fat Dairy May Help Fight
Hypertension

Researchers funded by the National Heart, Lung and Blood Institute may have found another way in which "milk does a body good." Their new study, published in *Hypertension,* suggests that milk and other dairy products can help combat high blood pressure—as long as the dairy is low in saturated fat.

The researchers used data in food questionnaires from 4,797 men (45%) and women, average age 52, participating in the Family Heart Study. Participants were divided into four groups based on their daily dairy intake; the highest dairy group consumed three or more servings daily, while the lowest consumed less than half a serving of dairy a day. Those in the highest-dairy group averaged systolic blood pressure 2.6 millimeters of mercury lower than the group consuming the least amount of dairy products. (Systolic blood pressure is the first number in a blood-pressure measurement, a test of pressure in the arteries when the left ventricle of the heart contracts to push blood through the body.)

Next, however, researchers divided the groups by those who ate below the average amount of saturated fat and those who ate above that amount. Because of the study's methodology, it wasn't possible to directly group participants by their consumption of low-fat dairy, only by overall saturated-fat intake from all sources, including dairy. When fat intake was taken into account, only the high-dairy consumers who *also* had low saturated-fat intake saw a benefit. Among all those consuming lower amounts of saturated fat, people who also ate or drank the most dairy products had a 54% lower odds of hypertension than those with the least dairy intake.

The researchers caution that the cross-sectional design of the study limits the ability to draw a causal relationship between dairy consumption and blood pressure. But Luc Djoussé, MD, MPH, DSc, lead author of the study and an associate epidemiologist at Brigham and Women's Hospital in Boston, says the evidence certainly suggests that low-fat dairy may help against hypertension.

"Our data showed that dairy consumption is inversely associated with prevalent high blood pressure and resting systolic blood pressure, mainly among individuals consuming less saturated fat and independent of the amount of dietary calcium," Dr. Djoussé says. "It is possible that nutrients other than calcium found in dairy products may be responsible for these findings.

"Dairy products, such as cheese, yogurt and milk, are excellent sources of calcium," he goes on. "However, some dairy products also contain substantial amounts of saturated fat, which might offset some of the beneficial effects of dairy products. In this study, magnesium and potassium intake was associated with lower blood pressure, but calcium was not."

Some 65 million Americans suffer from hypertension, which is a major risk factor for stroke, heart attack, kidney failure and heart failure.

To learn more: *Hypertension,* journal of the American Heart Association, August 2006; abstract at <hyper.ahajournals.org/cgi/content/abstract/01.HYP.0000229668.73501.e8v1>.

More Reasons to Eat Your Fruits & Vegetables
Getting More Protein from Plants May Lower Blood Pressure

People who consume regular daily portions of vegetables, whole grains and fruit tend to have healthier blood pressure levels than their more carnivorous peers, according to a new British study. The findings bolster recommendations that adults eat more plant-based foods for the sake of their cardiovascular health.

The study, published in the *Archives of Internal Medicine*, found that among nearly 4,700 middle-aged adults in four countries, those who ate more vegetable protein tended to have lower blood pressure. The apparent benefit was independent of other factors, such as exercise, sodium intake and body weight, according to Paul Elliott, MB, PhD, of Imperial College in London, the study's lead author. Elliott added that the findings lend support to recommendations to eat more plant-based foods.

The International Study on Macronutrients and Blood Pressure (INTERMAP) Cooperative Research Group recruited 1,145 participants from Japan, 839 from China, 501 from England and 2,195 from the US. Blood pressure was measured at four visits over three- to six-week intervals. At each visit the participants completed detailed diaries describing total food intake over the previous 24 hours. Urine specimens were collected at the first and third examinations.

Overall, the study found, average blood pressure levels dipped as vegetable protein intake increased. The opposite was true of animal protein intake. Participants for whom vegetable protein represented about 9% of total caloric intake had systolic blood pressures that were on average 2.14 mm Hg lower and diastolic pressures that were 1.35 mm Hg lower than those whose diets were not so rich in vegetable protein. Even after adjusting for height and weight, the differences were still significant; systolic pressure averaged 1.11 mm Hg lower and diastolic pressure was 0.71 mm Hg lower.

Blood pressure above optimal (120/80 mmHg) has been established as a major cardiovascular disease risk factor. The Dietary Approaches to Stop Hypertension, or DASH, Eating Plan, considered the best diet against high blood pressure, is low in sodium and fat, and emphasizes low-fat dairy, fruits and vegetables. The INTERMAP findings on vegetable protein underscore the effectiveness of that element of the DASH plan.

The study authors theorized that the association between vegetable protein and blood pressure may be explained by the action of amino acids. "We found significant differences in the amino acid content of diets predominating in vegetable protein compared with those predominating in animal protein," they wrote. That difference may explain the opposing effects of animal and vegetable protein.

By eating a significant amount of vegetable protein, people tend to take in high amounts of fiber and magnesium, which may account for at least some of the positive blood pressure effects. Vegetable proteins also contain specific amino acids—the "building blocks" of protein—that research suggests help control blood pressure.

Although a definitive explanation of the blood pressure benefits requires further study, the authors of the INTERMAP study concluded that it is "consistent with current recommendations that a diet high in vegetable products be part of a healthy lifestyle for prevention of high blood pressure and related chronic diseases."

To learn more: *Archives of Internal Medicine*, Jan. 9, 2006. Free abstract at
<archinte.ama-assn.org/ cgi/content/abstract/166/1/79>.
American Heart Association–High Blood Pressure
<www.americanheart.org/presenter.jhtml?identifier=2114>.

Hit the Sack to Help Avoid Hypertension

Getting too little sleep can lead to worse woes than bags under your eyes. A new study published in the American Heart Association journal *Hypertension* identifies sleeplessness as a significant risk factor for high blood pressure.

"It's been known for a long time that sleep disorders are associated with hypertension," says James E. Gangwisch, PhD, lead author of the study and a postdoctoral fellow at the Columbia University Medical Center, "but that could be for reasons besides not getting enough sleep. This is the first study that shows a relationship between short sleep duration itself and high blood pressure."

Researchers analyzed data from the National Health and Nutrition Examination Survey (NHANES) on 4,810 participants over 10 years. Those ages 32 to 59 who got five hours or less of sleep a night were more than twice as likely to develop hypertension than those who got the recommended norm of seven to eight hours. A significant difference remained even after controlling for known hypertension risk factors.

But still more sleep wasn't better: People who got nine hours or more of sleep were not significantly less likely to have high blood pressure than those who slept seven to eight hours, the study found.

While many factors contribute to high blood pressure—most notably obesity—lack of sleep appears to be an independent cause. Normally during sleep your heart rate and blood pressure are lower. In people deprived of sleep over a long period of time, however, the average work done by the heart increases, and that can lead to irreversible changes in the heart and blood vessels.

Gangwisch says the study's main message is clear: "A good night's sleep is very important for good health."

To learn more: *Hypertension,* published online before print
<hyper.ahajournals.org/cgi/content/ abstract/47/5/833>.

The Skinny on Fats

New Labeling Helps You Avoid Trans Fat

*But trans fats still lurk in fried foods, baked goods—
and butter's no better.*

After investing 30,000 hours in research and testing, Kraft Foods introduced an Oreo cookie that contains no trans fat. The company, like other food manufacturers, scrambled to meet a Food and Drug Administration (FDA) deadline adding trans fats to Nutrition Facts labels: All packaged foods with a half-gram or more of trans fat per serving must now fess up.

Trans fats, containing trans-fatty acids and typically labeled as "hydrogenated" oils, have been widely used in baking and frying because of their physical properties. Trans fats are formed when hydrogen is added to liquid oils—primarily soybean oil—which not only solidifies the oil but also makes it resist going rancid and degrading with reheating. Trans fats were also once touted as a cheap and apparently healthy alternative to butter and other animal fats.

But in 1990 Dutch researchers showed that trans fats increase LDL ("bad") cholesterol levels while decreasing HDL ("good") cholesterol. In 2002, the Institute of Medicine of the National Academy of Sciences advised that diets should minimize trans fat intake. When the FDA set its labeling requirement for January 2006, the rush to banish trans fat was on. At the height of trans-fat hysteria, New York City health commissioner Thomas Frieden, MD,

Nutrition Facts

Serving Size 1 cup (228g)
Servings Per Container 2

Amount Per Serving

Calories 260   Calories from Fat 120

	% Daily Value*
Total Fat 13g	**20%**
Saturated Fat 5g	**25%**
Trans Fat 2g	
Cholesterol 30mg	**10%**
Sodium 660mg	**28%**
Total Carbohydrate 31g	**10%**
Dietary Fiber 0g	**0%**
Sugars 5g	
Protein 5g	

Vitamin A 4%	•	Vitamin C 2%
Calcium 15%	•	Iron 4%

* Percent Daily Values are based on a 2,000 calorie diet. Your Daily Values may be higher or lower depending on your calorie needs:

	Calories:	2,000	2,500
Total Fat	Less than	65g	80g
Sat Fat	Less than	20g	25g
Cholesterol	Less than	300mg	300mg
Sodium	Less than	2,400mg	2,400mg
Total Carbohydrate		300g	375g
Dietary Fiber		25g	30g

Calories per gram:
Fat 9   •   Carbohydrate 4   •   Protein 4

called on restaurants to abandon hydrogenated fats, inaccurately likening them to toxic substances such as asbestos and lead.

The good news is that thousands of products, ranging from Oreo cookies to Triscuits crackers, are indeed shedding their trans fat. Now a glance at the label will identify those that haven't gotten with the program.

The bad news, however, is that America's $476 billion restaurant industry remains addicted to trans fats. And, even with zero trans fat, Oreo cookies still aren't exactly health food.

Fast-food chains, heavily reliant on frying, have been the slowest to kick the trans-fat habit. McDonald's, which switched from beef tallow to partially hydrogenated soybean oil in 1990, promised back in September 2002 to change its oil again. But it still hasn't delivered on that promise, and recently settled a lawsuit for $8.5 million for inadequately publicizing the delay. A Burger King spokesperson says trans fats have "never been an issue" with its customers.

For now, your best strategy to avoid trans fats—and, just as important, saturated fats—when eating out is to skip the fried foods. A large order of fries typically contains six grams of trans fat. Also beware of takeaway baked goods such as doughnuts. And, of course, check the new labels on commercially baked products like Oreos.

But, whether eating out or buying packaged foods, don't think that simply avoiding trans fat makes for a healthful choice. Some anti-trans fat crusaders have gone overboard in what *The New York Times* calls "the panic du jour"—going so far as to claim that switching to butter, palm oil or anything else would be an improvement over the dreaded trans fats.

The science doesn't back up that extreme position, however. Trans fat is no worse for your health than saturated fat, according to the National Academy of Sciences, National Heart, Lung and Blood Institute (NHLBI), Department of Health and Human Services and the FDA. In fact, James Cleeman, MD, coordinator of the NHLBI's National Cholesterol Education Program, told the *Times*, "What's Public Enemy No. 1 with respect to cholesterol raising? From a dietary standpoint, it's saturated fat."

"Don't switch from trans fat to saturated fat," advises Alice H. Lichtenstein, DSc, Stanley N. Gershoff Professor at Tufts' Friedman School of Nutrition Science and Policy. "The aim should be to minimize the intake of *both*. And remember that the bottom line is still total caloric intake."

So when you study the new Nutrition Facts labels, don't just look for a zero on the trans-fat line. (You'll notice that no percentage accompanies the trans-fat number when a product does have more than a half-gram per serving, since there is no Daily Value for trans fat.) Take a gander at the line above it, too: How much saturated fat are you getting per serving? And don't forget the top line, calories, whatever their source; if your caloric intake exceeds that burned in physical activity, you'll put on the pounds.

The American Heart Association (AHA) recommends a diet rich in fruits and vegetables, whole grains, low- and non-fat dairy products, legumes and fish. Lichtenstein, who chairs the AHA's nutrition committee, says, "What Americans need to do is focus on overall lifestyle patterns, move around more, and eat a healthy diet."

Sorry, that doesn't mean Oreo cookies—even those labeled zero trans fat.

To learn more: FDA Questions and Answers About Trans Fat Nutrition Labeling
<www.cfsan.fda.gov/~dms/qatrans2.html>

How Much Trans Fat Is Too Much? Almost Any

Keeping trans fatty acids out of your diet got easier in January 2006 when the US Food and Drug Administration (FDA) mandated labeling of foods containing more than 500 milligrams of trans fat per serving. Now a new review of the scientific literature on trans fats' health effects shows just how important it is to minimize your intake.

The report, published in the *New England Journal of Medicine*, cautioned that the trans fat problem hasn't been solved by the latest labeling rules. Consumers must still heed those food labels, and trans fats remain popular with restaurants and makers of packaged baked goods. Lead author Daniel Mozaffarian, MD, of the Harvard School of Public Health, said that the health risk of trans fats are still far more serious than those of contaminants or pesticide residue in foods.

In fact, the reviewers concluded that, on a per-calorie basis, trans fats increase the risk of coronary heart disease (CHD) more than any other micronutrient. Even at levels as low as 1-3% of total calorie consumption, trans fats were linked with significantly higher risk. In a meta-analysis of results from four prospective cohort studies totaling nearly 140,000 subjects, the review found that an increase of just 2% in caloric intake of trans fats was associated with a 23% higher risk of CHD. The authors also cited a large, community-based, case-control study that linked higher levels of trans fats to a 47% increased risk of sudden cardiac death.

The effects of trans-fat consumption were seen most dramatically in serum lipids—the levels of substances such as cholesterol in the blood. As have previous studies that helped lead to the FDA rule, the review concluded that trans fats not only raise levels of the "bad" LDL cholesterol, but also lower levels of the "good" HDL cholesterol. Trans-fat consumption also increases the proportion of total cholesterol to HDL cholesterol—a key predictor of heart risk.

Only in the case of diabetes was the evidence for trans fats' risky role somewhat ambiguous. Two of the studies examined failed to find a link between trans-fat consumption and diabetes, although a third study did show a positive association.

The reviewers estimated that 10-19% of CHD events in the US could be averted by reducing Americans' consumption of trans fats—up to 228,000 coronary events annually.

Because trans fats seem to elevate risk at intake levels as low as 20-60 calories a day (in a 2,000-calorie diet), the reviewers concluded, "complete or near-complete avoidance of industrially produced trans fats may be necessary to avoid adverse effects and would be prudent to minimize health risks."

> # What Makes Fat "Trans"?
>
> Trans fatty acids are created when hydrogen is added to the molecules of an ordinary liquid vegetable oil. That process makes these "partially hydrogenated" fats solid or semisolid at room temperature, as in margarines and the fats used in many commercial baked goods and restaurant deep-frying. Manufacturers and restaurants like partially hydrogenated vegetable oils because of their long shelf life, "buttery" taste and texture, and stability for deep-frying.

To learn more: *New England Journal of Medicine*, April 13, 2006.

Restaurant Trans-Fat Ban Cooks Up Controversy

Less than a year after the Food and Drug Administration (FDA) began requiring labeling of trans fat in supermarket foods, consumer advocates have declared war on trans fat in restaurants. The New York City Board of Health voted unanimously to consider banning all but a minute amount of trans fat in food served at the city's 20,000 restaurants. Days after the New York vote, the World Health Organization (WHO) recommended that governments worldwide move to phase out trans fats if labeling alone doesn't lead to significant reductions.

The city of Chicago is weighing its own regulations on restaurant trans fat. Canada, the first nation to mandate trans-fat labeling, may follow with a nationwide ban. To date, the only country to enact a ban is Denmark, which two years ago outlawed foods containing more than 2% trans fats.

Research has implicated trans fat as being especially heart-unhealthy, increasing LDL ("bad") cholesterol while reducing HDL ("good") cholesterol levels. Certain restaurant food can be particularly high in trans fats. Places that fry a lot of food prefer "hydrogenated" oil because it can be used longer. This process of adding hydrogen improves shelf life, makes oil solid

McDonald's Fries Found Trans-Fattier

You probably already knew that McDonald's French fries aren't health food. But until recently, not even the fast-food giant knew just how much trans fat was in its fries. Citing the results of an improved testing method, McDonald's announced that its fries contain one-third more trans fat than previously calculated: eight grams rather than six, with total fat jumping to 30 grams from 25. Trans fats have been shown to contribute to heart disease by increasing LDL ("bad") cholesterol levels while decreasing HDL ("good") cholesterol. (See the January 2006 Healthletter.) McDonald's made the disclosure while rolling out new food packaging that includes nutritional facts.

To learn more: McDonald's Nutrition Information
<www.mcdonalds.com/usa/eat/ nutrition_info.html>.

or semisolid at room temperature, gives it a more "buttery" taste and texture—and creates trans-fatty acids.

Turning up the heat on menus

Harvard nutrition researcher Walter Willett, MD, DrPH, has calculated that one-third to one-half of the typical American's trans-fat consumption comes from restaurants. Dr. Willett estimated that New York City's proposed ban would prevent 500 deaths annually.

"Like lead paint, artificial trans fat is invisible and dangerous, and it can be replaced," said New York City Health Commissioner Thomas R. Frieden. "No one will miss it when it is gone."

The city regulations are aimed not only at corner delis but at national restaurant chains—which legal experts predict will spark court challenges. McDonald's has promised to change its French-fry oil, but that switch is still pending as the fast-food giant struggles to maintain flavor. Similarly, Burger King says it has tested alternative oils but met consumer taste resistance. Applebee's, the US' biggest casual-dining chain, has reduced trans fats in desserts and baked goods, but not the rest of its menu.

Other restaurant chains have been more aggressive in cutting trans fat, including Wendy's, Panera Bread Co., Ruby Tuesday, California Pizza Kitchen and Legal Sea Food, according to an analysis by the *Wall Street Journal*. KFC recently announced it would stop using trans fats.

How big a benefit?

But the benefits of banning trans fat in restaurants may not be as dramatic as advocates hope. "It's no panacea," cautions Alice H. Lichtenstein, DSc, director of the Cardiovascular Nutrition Laboratory at Tufts' Jean

Mayer USDA Human Nutrition Research Center on Aging (HNRCA). "Clearly we do not need trans-fatty acids; they are not essential nutrients, as are vitamins and minerals, and there is no benefit to having them in the diet. However, we are still not tackling the 'big giant' in the room—too many calories and too little activity."

Lichtenstein dismisses a commonly cited estimate that the average American consumes 2.6% of calories from trans fat—that's old data, she says. "Besides, averages do not matter that much. What matters is that there are some people with low intakes and some people with very high intakes; obviously, people at the high end should decrease intake."

In research at the HNRCA, Lichtenstein and colleagues did confirm a "linear" relationship between trans-fat intake and LDL cholesterol: The more trans fat subjects consumed, the worse their LDL levels.

But the alternatives to trans fat may not be much better. New York's health office has even urged restaurants to switch to butter—a major source of saturated fat, as are palm oil and coconut oil, popular baking alternatives. Saturated fat is the leading culprit in unhealthy cholesterol levels.

The average consumer's best bet when eating out remains smart scrutiny of restaurant menus. Minimize intake of commercially

Trans fat in popular restaurant items:

- McDonald's Big Mac–1.5 grams
- McDonald's Sausage Biscuit with Egg–5 grams
- Burger King medium French fries–4.5 grams
- Burger King French Toast Sticks (5 pieces)–4.5 grams
- Wendy's Homestyle Chicken Strips (3 pieces)–zero grams
- Wendy's medium French fries–0.5 grams
- Dunkin' Donuts Glazed Donut–4 grams
- Panera Bread Asiago Roast Beef Sandwich–1 gram

fried foods and baked goods because, unless otherwise stated, they are high in trans fat. But also watch out for saturated fat, the greasy fat in meats and cheese. Load up instead on vegetables (not fried), fruits and whole grains.

And remember that "big giant" in the room. Indeed, Lichtenstein points to another proposed New York City health regulation as being at least as important as the headline-grabbing trans-fat ban: Requiring posting the calorie content of food in restaurants as prominently as the price. "Because we eat such a large amount of food that is prepared outside the home," she says, "this could have a tremendous impact on caloric intake where the problem starts—at the point of purchase."

Should You Give Eggs a Second Chance?

It's no wonder Americans are at a loss when it comes to deciding whether to eat eggs, once touted as "nature's perfect food." Low-carb eating plans that feature high-protein eggs for breakfast clash with well-publicized concerns over elevated cholesterol levels and increased risk of heart disease.

But more recent studies and revised recommendations may lift the cloud over eggs, revealing a sunny-side-up lining to "the incredible, edible egg" after all.

For much of the past 40 years, the public has been warned away from eggs because of heart disease risk. Unhealthy serum cholesterol levels have, after all, been conclusively linked to increased risk of cardiovascular disease (CVD) and eggs are relatively high in dietary cholesterol.

But guidelines to limit egg consumption to no more than one egg a week have been revisited and considered too strict by some experts, considering eggs' other nutritional benefits. Eggs provide a number of heart-healthy nutrients, such as folate, vitamins E and B12, omega-3 and omega-6 fatty acids, as well as antioxidants such as lutein, which is important for good eye health.

Increasing understanding about the causes of high LDL cholesterol levels has also helped unscramble the difference between cholesterol in the blood and cholesterol in food. That's made the humble egg no longer public enemy number-one in the battle against heart disease.

Dietary vs. Serum Cholesterol

Cholesterol is made naturally in the body of all animals and humans. It is necessary for the production of hormones and vitamin D, and to keep cell walls healthy. The liver makes most of the cholesterol needed by the human body, so you shouldn't have to worry about getting "enough" from your food.

Dietary cholesterol is found in animal foods, such as meat, fish, poultry, milk products and, of course, eggs. While the cholesterol in food can raise your blood cholesterol levels—known as "serum cholesterol"—scientists now know that consuming saturated fat and trans fat (hydrogenated fat) generally contributes more to unhealthy serum-cholesterol levels.

You probably already know that there are two main types of serum cholesterol: HDL and LDL. The "good" HDL cholesterol can reduce the buildup of plaque on artery walls; high serum HDL levels are associated with a lower risk of heart disease. The "bad" LDL cholesterol can contribute to a buildup of plaque in the arteries, and high serum LDL levels are linked to heart disease.

Much of the past panic over egg consumption comes from the multiple uses of the term "cholesterol" and confusion between cholesterol in food and unhealthy cholesterol levels in the blood. Dietary cholesterol does not automatically become blood cholesterol when you eat it.

That doesn't mean you can forget about cholesterol on those nutrition labels or gobble eggs like a fox in the proverbial henhouse. But it is true that your fight against cardiovascular disease probably should start with sharply reducing saturated and trans fat and increasing physical activity—not by tossing out all the eggs in your refrigerator.

Eggs and Your Heart

Some research has even questioned the connection between egg consumption and cardiovascular disease. A study by the Food and Nutrition Database Research Center at Michigan State University, published in the *Journal of the American College of Nutrition* in 2000, showed that risk of CVD in men and women did not increase with increasing egg consumption. In fact, quite the opposite!

The study's more than 27,000 subjects were participants in the National Health and Nutritional Examination Survey (NHANES) who reported their egg-eating habits as part of a 24-hour-recall food diary. Excluded from the study were subjects with unreliable dietary recall records, pregnant and lactating women, those taking cholesterol-lowering drugs or medications for unspecified heart disease, and those who consumed only the whites of eggs or egg-white commercial products, such as Egg-Beaters. Serum cholesterol data from subjects who reported changing their diet in the past year due to high serum cholesterol level also were not included. In contrast to earlier studies that fed subjects dehydrated egg yolks, the Michigan State University study compared consumers and non-consumers of actual whole eggs.

Focusing on the nutritional benefits of eggs, as well as dietary versus serum cholesterol levels, the study suggested that benefits to the heart from the nutrients found in whole eggs (such as polyunsaturated fat, folate and vitamins A and E) actually may outweigh the potentially adverse effects of their cholesterol. In the published results, researchers Won O. Song, PhD, MPH, RD, and Jean M. Kerver, MS, RD, asserted that eggs make important nutritional contributions to the American diet, and that relatively frequent egg consumption did not contribute negatively to serum cholesterol levels.

Their findings indicated that the egg consumers actually had lower serum cholesterol levels than those subjects who abstained from eggs. While men who ate two to three eggs per week had slightly lower levels than men who consumed four eggs or more per week, both groups had lower serum cholesterol levels than those who abstained completely. And in women, those who ate four or more eggs per week had the lowest levels of all.

Song and Kerver concluded, "Our work repudiates the hypothesis that increased egg consumption leads to increased serum cholesterol concentrations, and also adds to the growing body of literature which supports the nutritional benefits of eggs." Short of labeling eggs as "medicinal," the researchers cautioned, "although our results suggest that higher egg consumption is associated with lower serum cholesterol, this study should not be used as a basis for recommending higher egg consumption for regulation of serum cholesterol."

Dietary Cholesterol, By the Numbers

Such findings in recent years have caused some experts to retreat from the one-egg-a-week limit. But that doesn't mean you should stop watching dietary cholesterol altogether. Both the American Heart Association and the National Heart, Lung and Blood Institute's National Cholesterol Education Program advise limiting dietary cholesterol to an average of 300 milligrams a day for healthy people, and around 200 milligrams per day for those who already have heart disease.

One egg yolk, where the cholesterol in eggs resides, contains about 215 milligrams of cholesterol. So, theoretically, healthy people could get away with eating an egg a day—if you're not getting much cholesterol from other dietary sources. Eat that single egg for breakfast with a traditional slice of buttered toast and two strips of bacon, though, and you're already at almost 250 milligrams of cholesterol—and the day's barely started. (Of course, you also need to control intake of saturated fat.) Many baked dishes also contain eggs, and these "hidden" eggs can quickly boost your dietary-cholesterol intake.

So Ernst J. Schaefer, MD, senior scientist in the Lipids Metabolism Laboratory at Tufts' Jean Mayer USDA Human Nutrition Research Center on Aging and a professor at the Friedman School of Nutrition Science and Policy, urges going slowly about advocating increased egg consumption. He points out that recent egg-cholesterol studies used the subjects' self-reported food diaries as proof of their egg consumption, rather than the subjects being fed a strictly administered regimen.

"In carefully controlled studies, we do see some elevation of cholesterol levels with increased egg consumption," Dr. Schaefer says. In controlled diet studies he did together with Alice H. Lichtenstein, DSc, Stanley N. Gershoff Professor of Nutrition at Tufts, just one and a half eggs daily (about 320 milligrams of cholesterol) raised the bad LDL cholesterol by

Nutrition Facts

Serving Size 1 egg (50g)
Serving per Container 12

Amount Per Serving

Calories 70   Calories from Fat 40

	% Daily Value*
Total Fat 4.5g	7%
Saturated Fat 1.5g	8%
Polyunsaturated Fat .5g	
Monounsaturated Fat 2.0g	
Cholesterol 215mg	71%
Sodium 65mg	3%
Potassium 60mg	2%
Total Carbohydrate 1g	0%
Protein 6g	10%

Vitamin A 6% · Vitamin C 0%
Calcium 2% · Iron 4% · Thiamin 2%
Riboflavin 15% · Vitamin B-6 4%
Folate 6% · Vitamin B-12 8%
Phosphorus 8% · Zinc 4%

Not a significant source of Dietary Fiber or Sugars.

*Percent Daily Values are based on a 2,000 calorie diet. Your daily values may be higher or lower depending on your calorie needs.

	Calories	2,000	2,500
Total Fat	Less than	65g	80g
Sat Fat	Less than	20g	25g
Cholesterol	Less than	300mg	300mg
Sodium	Less than	2,400mg	2,400mg
Potassium		3,500mg	3,500mg
Total Carbohydrate		300g	375g
Dietary Fiber		25g	30g
Protein		50g	65g

Calories per gram
Fat 9 · Carbohydrate 4 · Protein 4

about 10% in middle-aged and elderly subjects who already had above-average LDL levels.

"Although clearly not as strong a factor as saturated fat," Lichtenstein adds, "hundreds of studies including our own have shown that adding eggs/cholesterol to someone's diet increases serum cholesterol in susceptible individuals."

Dr. Schaefer also wonders about "the rest of the day," when people are sure to consume additional dietary cholesterol. "If people in the elevated risk category are going to eat an egg, that's their whole day's allotment. Are they then not going to ever eat a hamburger, or even have some dressing on their salad?" he asks. "I tell people to use Egg-Beaters (instead of eggs). They have no saturated fat, are relatively inexpensive, they taste great and have the essential amino acids of (whole) eggs."

Dr. Schaefer suggests that the bio-available nutrients in spinach would make up for the nutritional components sacrificed by omitting the eggs' yolks. He advises, "An Egg-Beater spinach omelet could be the perfect answer."

Handle with Care

Another rap against eggs in recent years has nothing to do with their nutritional value—it's the question of food safety. It's true, raw eggs can harbor dangerous bacteria such as salmonella. Even the industry-boosting American Egg Board concedes, "The nutrients that make eggs a high-quality food for humans are also a good growth medium for bacteria." Although the inside of an egg was once considered essentially sterile, in recent years the Salmonella enteritidis bacteria has been found in eggs. The incidence of salmonella in eggs remains extremely rare, however—estimated at 1 in every 20,000 eggs.

Still, better safe than sorry when it comes to food safety and eggs. Here are some tips on egg safety and healthy egg preparation from the 2005 Dietary Guidelines for Americans and the US Food and Drug Administration Center for Food Safety and Applied Nutrition:

• Use only properly refrigerated, clean, sound-shelled, fresh, grade AA or A eggs.

• Consider pasteurized egg products, including the new pasteurized-in-the-shell eggs.

• Store eggs in the carton on a shelf in the refrigerator to ensure freshness.

• Egg shell and yolk color may vary, but color has nothing to do with egg quality, flavor or nutritive value.

• Poach eggs instead of frying to cut back on fat, or use non-stick pans or non-stick vegetable pan spray.

• Serve egg dishes promptly or keep them refrigerated. Remember the

Two-Hour Rule: Don't leave perishables out at room temperature for more than two hours. Bacteria love to grow in protein-rich foods such as egg dishes.

• Whether you like your breakfast eggs scrambled or fried, always cook eggs until the yolks and whites are firm.

• Tasting is tempting, but licking a spoon or tasting raw cookie dough from a mixing bowl can be risky. Bacteria could be lurking in the raw eggs.

• Cook cheesecakes and egg dishes to an internal temperature of at least 160 degrees Fahrenheit. Use a food thermometer to check.

It's up to you and your doctor whether and how much to incorporate eggs into your diet. But with moderation and smart food-safety steps, you can occasionally enjoy "nature's perfect food" without fear.

To learn more: *Journal of the American College of Nutrition*, October 2000; free text online at <www.jacn.org/cgi/content/full/19/suppl_5/556S>. FDA "Playing It Safe with Eggs" <www.foodsafety.gov/~fsg/fs-eggs3.html>. American Egg Board <www.aeb.org>.

Behind the Headlines on Low-Fat Diet Study

Despite the headlines, the latest findings on dietary fat don't mean you should give up on watching the fat in your food. True, the widely reported $415 million government study, the Women's Health Initiative (WHI) Dietary Modification Trial, generally failed to find benefits from a low-fat diet against breast and colon cancer or cardiovascular disease. But that doesn't mean, as a *New York Times* editorial opined, "The more we learn about nutrition, the less we seem to know."

"This was a carefully done and well carried out study that was badly served by the press," says *Healthletter* editor Irwin H. Rosenberg, MD, University Professor at Tufts' Friedman School of Nutrition Science and Policy. "The damage done to efforts to persuade people to take responsibility in picking their diets is huge. If the subtext is that diet has nothing to do with health and disease, that's a dangerous and irresponsible message."

The real lesson here, according to Dr. Rosenberg, is the limitation of any one study—even a controlled clinical trial, considered the "gold standard" of nutrition research. And this was certainly a large-scale study: Researchers at 40 US clinical centers involved 48,835 postmenopausal women, ages 50 to 79, in three trials of the effects of reducing total dietary fat. Those assigned to the intervention group—19,541 women—were given behavior modification with a goal of reducing fat intake to 20% of calories, while increasing fruits and vegetables to at least five daily servings and grains to six servings.

The results were published in three articles in the *Journal of the American Medical Association* (JAMA). Researchers found no significant difference between women on the low-fat diet and a control group in risk of breast or colon cancer or cardiovascular disease. "The results, of course, are somewhat disappointing," study co-authors JoAnn Manson, MD, DrPH, chief of preventive medicine at Harvard's Brigham and Women's Hospital, told the Associated Press. "We would have liked this dietary intervention to have a major impact on health."

But Dr. Manson cautioned, "These results do not suggest that people have carte blanche to eat fatty foods without health problems."

Robert H. Eckel, MD, president of the American Heart Association (AHA), agrees: "It would be easy to misinterpret the results of this study, and it is important that we get it right. Reducing the risk of cardiovascular disease is about following an integrated lifestyle program, rather than concentrating solely on dietary composition."

To understand why not all experts view this study as the final or even definitive word on fat and health, it helps to know a little about the genesis of the research. A number of animal tests and observational studies on humans had suggested a link between total fat intake and cancer risk, especially breast cancer. Although many people assume cutting fat can fight cancer, the idea has actually been very controversial in the medical community, says Michael Thun, MD, vice president of epidemiology for the American Cancer Society. Since this WHI study began, he adds, there's been greater evidence that being overweight or obese is much more important to cancer risk than total fat intake.

Although researchers also looked at heart disease, "by the time the study was initiated, we already knew that for heart disease at least the evidence was much more strongly related to saturated fat than to total fat," Dr. Rosenberg points out. The study did not specifically target saturated fat—which the AHA recommends limiting to 10% of total calories for healthy people—or differentiate between total fat and heart-healthier choices such as monounsaturated or polyunsaturated fat. The federal dietary guidelines released since the study's inception don't focus on total fat, but instead advise limiting both saturated fat and trans fat.

The women in the study also failed to achieve their fat-cutting goals: They got down to 24% in the first year, then slid to 29% as the study went on.

And although participants were studied for an average of 8.1 years, even that may not be long enough, Dr. Rosenberg says: "You're looking at conditions that may take decades in some cases to develop."

Finally, the research did discover some positive results: On breast cancer, women consuming the most fat prior to the study and those at high risk—testing positive for the estrogen receptor and negative for the progesterone receptor—showed significant benefits. Researchers found a small but statistically significant reduction in levels of LDL ("bad" cholesterol) and diastolic blood pressure. And, as current thinking would suggest, women with lower consumption of saturated and trans fats and more fruits and vegetables did see a trend toward reduced heart disease risk.

Nonetheless, the results may help burst the low-fat bubble that led food marketers to label 12.8% of new products released last year as low-fat or fat-free. Oversimplifying nutritional advice to merely "avoid fat" may have been a mistake in the first place, Dr. Rosenberg observes. "It underestimated the ability of the American public to hear a more complex nutritional message."

To learn more: *Journal of the American Medical Association*, Feb. 8, 2006. Free abstracts at <jama.ama-assn.org/content/vol295/issue6/ index.dtl>.
American Heart Association <www.americanheart.org/presenter.jhtml?identifier=4582>.
American Cancer Society <www.cancer.org/docroot/ NWS/nws_0.asp>.

Coconut oil:
"miracle" or simply saturated fat?

Q For years I was under the impression that fats that are solid at room temperature should be avoided or consumed sparingly. Could you explain why Extra Virgin Coconut Oil is sold in health-food stores? I understand that it has no cholesterol, but the saturated fat and the solid-at-room-temperature property concern me. Could you tell me more about coconut oil in regard to healthful nutrition?

A The health-food stores you frequent have no doubt been swayed by popular books touting "the coconut oil miracle," "the healing miracle of coconut oil" and "Virgin Coconut Oil: How It Has Changed People's Lives, and How It Can Change Yours!" Despite the success of such titles, according to Alice H. Lichtenstein, DSc, Gershoff Professor of nutrition science and policy at Tufts' Friedman School, "To my knowledge there is no scientific basis to back these claims." She adds, "Coconut oil is rich in saturated fat, hence the recommendation is to restrict intake." Saturated fat, whether in "miraculous" coconut oil or ordinary butter, has been shown to contribute to heart disease. According to the USDA Nutrient Data Laboratory, one tablespoon of coconut oil contains 11.7 grams of saturated fat. And don't forget that all fats are high in calories—that tablespoon of coconut oil adds 117 calories your body must burn off to avoid gaining weight.

Grapeseed oil

Q Often you extol the virtues of canola and olive oils, but grapeseed oil is never mentioned. I have read that it lowers LDL and raises HDL—unlike any other oils available. It has less saturated fat than other commonly used oils. Since you never mention it, though, I wonder if there are negative health aspects that I should be aware of?

A The only negative aspect of grapeseed oil compared to other oils is that it tends to be more expensive and harder to find. It is among the lowest available oils in saturated fat, with only 10% (canola oil has the least at 7%). Grapeseed oil is also high in vitamin E, with more than canola or olive oil although less than safflower oil. From the cook's perspective, grapeseed oil is an excellent choice because of its high smoke point—about 420 degrees Fahrenheit (a temperature that will, however, destroy that vitamin E)—and light, "nutty" taste.

As an oil high in polyunsaturated fat (71%), grapeseed oil will tend to reduce dangerous LDL cholesterol a bit more than mostly monosaturated alternatives such as olive oil. But some studies have suggested that polyunsaturated fats may also lower the "good" HDL cholesterol at the same time. The claims that grapeseed oil actually raises HDL levels are based on two studies published in 1990, in the *Journal of Arteriosclerosis*, and 1993, in the *Journal of the American College of Cardiology*. Because grapeseed oil is far less common than other oils, its effects on health have not been as thoroughly studied, and these findings—more than a decade old—have not subsequently been confirmed by other research.

So, while you shouldn't expect miracles from grapeseed oil, it's a suitable alternative vegetable oil and a big improvement over cooking with fats that are solid at room temperature such as butter. But like all fats, grapeseed oil contains 120 calories per tablespoon, so use in moderation.

Spraying misinformation

Q A friend recently remarked that she was told by a dietician that when olive oil is sprayed from a can such as Pam and heated in a fry pan, it turns to trans fat. The friend was not sure if the same is true of spraying canola oil as well. I use this method of spraying the oil from a can every day and wonder if there is merit to this concern.

A Some bits of misinformation, like this one, simply refuse to die; instead they come back with a new twist. We've debunked this concern before as it relates to pouring olive oil for cooking. Don't worry—spraying the oil makes no difference in its potential to transform into trans fat, which has been shown to contribute to heart disease. While some trans fats occur naturally in animal products, by far the biggest dietary source is vegetable oil that has been "hydrogenated." This chemical process turns liquid vegetable oils into solids at room temperature, such as stick margarine and shortening. But you can't hydrogenate any oil in your home kitchen: The process requires adding hydrogen to the molecules of a vegetable oil, and uses hydrogen gas plus a metal catalyst, such as nickel.

The only danger from cooking spray, in fact, comes from spraying the oil onto a pan near an open flame. Always turn off a gas stove burner or move well away from a barbecue grill before spraying cooking oil.

Eating to Beat Cancer

Seeking Links Between
Diet and Colon Cancer

*Studies fail to find fiber benefits, implicate processed meat.
Plus: Good news on chicken?*

While dietary fiber has plenty of other benefits, it may not prevent colorectal cancer. On the other hand, eating a lot of processed meats—such as hot dogs, ham, bacon, sausage and lunch meats—probably does increase your risk of this cancer, which is second only to lung cancer as a cause of cancer deaths. But the good news is that—for reasons scientists can't yet explain—eating chicken seems to be associated with a reduced risk of colorectal cancer.

Those are the sometimes-surprising findings of two new studies of diet and the risk of cancer of the colon or rectum, which kills 56,000 Americans annually. The first study, an analysis of the combined data from 13 previous studies involving 725,628 men and women and ranging from six to 20 years, was published in the *Journal of the American Medical Association (JAMA)*. Close on its heels came the publication of a second study of 1,520 participants in two randomized trials, the Antioxidant Polyp Prevention Study and the Calcium Polyp Prevention Study, in the *American Journal of Gastroenterology*. All 1,520 subjects had a recent history of benign colorectal tumors called adenomas; the adenomas were removed, and patients got follow-up colonoscopies one and four years later.

The *JAMA* meta-analysis did find a significant benefit for fiber after adjusting only for subjects' ages. But after taking into account other dietary factors, such as folate intake, red-meat consumption and alcohol use, that benefit all but disappeared from the data. Contrary to some other findings on fiber and colorectal cancer, the conclusion was that the association was not statistically significant.

That's no reason to stop consuming fiber, however. The researchers—led by Yikyung Park, DSc, of the Harvard School of Public Health, now a visiting fellow at the National Cancer Institute—noted that benefits have been found for fiber from whole plants against an array of other disorders, including diabetes and heart disease.

"Colorectal cancer arguably has the most confusing association with fiber," noted John A. Baron, MD, of Dartmouth Medical School, in an accompanying editorial. Further research will be needed to sort out this confusion and the conflicting studies, Dr. Baron wrote.

The second new study, authored by Douglas J. Robertson, MD, MPH, also of the Dartmouth Medical School and of White River Junction VA Medical Center, was similarly discouraging about fiber's protective powers. Only a weak, non-significant association was found between fiber intake and reduced risk of recurrent adenomas, although a stronger benefit was seen against recurrence in the proximal colon. The strongest association with reduced risk was seen for fiber from vegetables and fruit and for fiber from grains.

On the flip side, subjects who ate the most processed meats had a 75% greater risk of advanced adenoma recurrence than those who ate little or no processed meat. The researchers fingered a possible increase in carcinogens in meat from salting, smoking or adding nitrates as the likely culprit.

The study found no added risk from consuming red meat, unlike some previous research, or fat.

Perhaps the most surprising result, however, was a beneficial association with eating chicken. The subjects who ate the most chicken had a 39% reduced risk of adenoma recurrence compared to the group consuming the least chicken.

"The mechanism by which poultry intake would independently reduce colorectal cancer incidence is not clearly delineated," the researchers wrote. "Poultry is a minor source of the nutrients selenium and calcium that have been associated with decreased risk for colorectal cancer."

In any case, they noted, the study suggests that some of the dietary guidance given to fight heart disease may also be good advice against colorectal cancer: Cut down on processed meats and include lean meat such as chicken (without the skin) in a balanced diet.

To learn more: *Journal of the American Medical Association*, Dec. 14, 2005; free abstract at <jama.ama-assn.org/cgi/content/abstract/ 294/22/2849>. *American Journal of Gastroenterology*, Dec. 2005; free abstract at <www.amjgastro.com>, click abstract for 2789. American Cancer Society <www.cancer.org/colonmd/pdfs/ ColonCancerFactSheet2005.DOC>.

Tea Time May Protect Against Ovarian Cancer

If you needed one more reason to begin a habit of drinking tea, the results of a new Swedish study might just push you over the edge and into the tea aisle of your grocery or health food store. Susanna C. Larsson, MSc, and colleagues reported in the *Archives of Internal Medicine* that middle-aged women who drink two or more cups of green or black tea every day may reduce their risk for invasive epithelial ovarian cancer by almost half.

The Karolinska Institute researchers studied 61,057 women ages 40 to 76 who completed a diet questionnaire and were then tracked for an average of 15.1 years. Women who consumed two or more cups of tea per day lowered their risk for ovarian cancer by 46%, with each additional cup lowering the risk by another 18%. The study found that even enjoying a spot of tea only occasionally offered some benefit: Those who drank less than one cup daily still reduced their risk somewhat when compared with women who rarely or never drank tea.

Tea contains antioxidant polyphenols, substances thought to block cell damage that can lead to cancer. Jeffrey Blumberg, PhD, a professor in Tufts' Friedman School of Nutrition Science and Policy, notes that the antioxidant capacity per cup is similar between green and black tea. You can think of tea as another serving of plant food, providing phytochemicals similar to those in fruits and vegetables, Blumberg says.

The results in the Swedish study may not be entirely due to tea, however, Julie Buring, DSc, of Harvard's Brigham and Women's Hospital cautioned in an Associated Press report. She noted the study also found that women who drank tea tended to be in better health, thanks to lifestyle habits. Indeed, the study's authors acknowledged that "the women who were regular tea drinkers were also those who ate more fruits and vegetables, were slimmer, and generally more health-conscious."

Still, Larsson and her team concluded that the dose-response relationship for tea consumption with ovarian cancer risk makes a strong case for the preventive properties of tea.

Ovarian cancer is the fourth leading cause of cancer death in women, diagnosed in more than 20,000 women in the US yearly. Its symptoms, including abdominal bloating, indigestion and urinary urgency, can be vague and mimic less serious conditions, making ovarian cancer difficult to detect early.

To learn more: *Archives of Internal Medicine*, Dec. 12, 2005; free abstract online at <archinte.ama-assn.org/cgi/content/short/165/22/2683>.

Increased Vitamin D Intake Recommended to Reduce Cancer Risks

A review of 63 observational studies of vitamin D and cancer concludes that boosting daily intake to 1,000 international units (IU) might reduce the risk of colon, ovarian, breast and possibly prostate cancer. That's more than the current Institute of Medicine recommendation for vitamin D, which ranges from 200-600 IU daily depending on age, though only half the safe upper limit set by the institute. Because it's difficult to get that much vitamin D from food alone, this target can likely be best achieved through supplements, according to study co-author Cedric F. Garland, DrPH, of the University of California.

"The cost of a daily dose of vitamin D3 (1,000 IU) is less than five cents, which could be balanced against the high human and economic costs of treating cancer attributable to insufficiency of vitamin D," the researchers wrote in the *American Journal of Public Health*. (This recommendation is not colored by the recent negative findings on vitamin D, calcium and bone benefits.)

According to Garland, vitamin D may ward off cancer by angiogenesis—inhibiting the growth of new blood vessels that allow cancer to thrive. Vitamin D can also enhance intercellular communication, "strengthening the inhibition of cancer cell growth that results from tight physical contact with adjacent cells within a tissue."

The researchers compared the number of positive versus negative studies for each type of cancer. Of 30 studies on colon cancer and vitamin D, 20 found a statistically significant benefit. Nine of 13 breast cancer studies reported a favorable association, as did five of seven ovarian cancer studies and half of 26 prostate cancer studies.

To learn more: *American Journal of Public Health*, February 2006. Free abstract at
<www.ajph.org/cgi/content/short/96/2/252>.

New Studies Boost Hopes for Vitamin D as Cancer Weapon

Vitamin D may not exactly be "the miracle vitamin," as a recent *Reader's Digest* breathlessly hyped it, but evidence of its health benefits does keep making headlines. Now, researchers have found that getting the daily adequate intake of vitamin D (400 IU) may reduce the risk of pancreatic cancer. The new study, in *Cancer Epidemiology Biomarkers & Prevention*, found a protective effect regardless of whether the vitamin D came from food, supplements or a combination.

"Because there is no effective screening for pancreatic cancer, identifying controllable risk factors for the disease is essential for developing strategies that can prevent cancer," said lead author Halcyon G. Skinner, PhD, currently at the University of Wisconsin School of Medicine and Public Health. "Vitamin D has shown a strong potential for preventing and treating prostate cancer, and areas with greater sunlight exposure have lower incidence and mortality for prostate, breast and colon cancers, leading us to investigate a role for vitamin D in pancreatic cancer risk."

Prevention is particularly important for pancreatic cancer, the US' fourth-leading cause of death from cancer, because it's rarely detected early enough to treat. Some 32,000 new cases are diagnosed annually, and only 5% of patients survive longer than five years.

The epidemiological cohort study analyzed data on 46,771 men ages 40 to 75 from the Health Professionals Follow-up Study and on 75,427 women ages 38 to 65 from the Nurses' Health Study who completed diet questionnaires. Over 16 years of follow-up, there were 365 cases of pancreatic cancer.

Compared with those in the lowest vitamin D-intake group (less than 150 IU daily), those getting 300 to 449 IU daily had 43% less risk of pancreatic cancer. Risk was also reduced, but not significantly different, for those at even higher vitamin D levels.

Further evidence of vitamin D's possible anti-cancer benefits comes from a second new study that suggests it may be associated with a slower progression of breast cancer. Researchers at Imperial College of London measured vitamin D levels in blood samples of 279 women with breast cancer. The study found that levels of vitamin D were lower in the 75 women with advanced breast cancer than in the 204 women with early-stage cancer.

Lead author Carlo Palmieri, MD, noted that the researchers don't know whether the low levels of vitamin D are a cause or a consequence of the cancer. But he points out, "There is in vitro, epidemiological and in vivo data to support the view that vitamin D has a role to play in the pathogenesis and progression of breast cancer.

"The next step in this research is to try and understand the potential causes and mechanisms underlying these differences and the precise consequences at a molecular level," Dr. Palmieri says.

To learn more: *Cancer Epidemiology Biomarkers & Prevention*, September 2006; abstract at <cebp.aacr-journals.org/cgi/content/abstract/15/9/1688>. *Journal of Clinical Pathology* online ahead of print, abstract at <jcp.bmjjournals.com/cgi/content/abstract/jcp.2006.042747v1>.

FDA Allows Watered-Down Tomato Claims vs. Cancer, Nixes Lycopene Claim

Tomatoes have plenty of nutritional benefits, but can eating tomatoes also fight cancer? Sort of. Maybe. It depends. That's how you might interpret the recent ruling by the US Food and Drug Administration (FDA), after two years of investigation, granting a "qualified health claim" for fresh, dried and canned tomatoes regarding four types of cancers. Even though the FDA allowed marketers to use some extremely watered-down language in their packaging, technically the ruling was a "partial denial." The tomato claims okayed by the FDA are so cautious, in fact, that companies such as H.J. Heinz probably won't put them on its products, though the claims will be used in customer communications.

The FDA also flatly rejected any cancer-benefits claim for dietary supplements containing lycopene, the antioxidant that gives tomatoes their red color. The agency found "no credible evidence" that lycopene—either in food or as a supplement—reduces cancer. American Longevity, a San Diego-based supplement maker that had petitioned the FDA, reacted angrily to the ruling and vowed to sue on First Amendment grounds.

The FDA's strongest endorsement of a health claim for tomatoes was against prostate cancer, where the agency cited "very limited and preliminary scientific research (that) suggests that eating one-half to one cup of tomatoes and/or tomato sauce a week may reduce the risk." But the agency cautioned, "There is very little scientific evidence supporting this claim."

While allowing qualified health claims for tomatoes against three other types of cancer, the FDA was even more lukewarm in its language. It's "unlikely that tomatoes reduce the risk" of gastric cancer, according to the agency, "highly uncertain" that tomatoes combat ovarian cancer, and "highly unlikely" that tomatoes help prevent pancreatic cancer.

F. Kerr Dow, PhD, vice president and chief technical officer for Heinz, nonetheless said the company, which had petitioned the FDA as part of the Lycopene Health Claim Coalition, was "very pleased that we finally got the FDA to come out and acknowledge the link" between tomato products and prostate cancer prevention. Dow conceded, however, that the ruling was "pretty complicated and not very inspiring."

In an interview with MedPage Today, Marion Nestle, PhD, a nutrition professor at New York University and author of books on the politics of food, said that in the face of legal challenges and industry pressure, the FDA began allowing qualified health claims that are "increasingly ridiculous." She called the new tomato claims "the height of ridiculous."

The controversy and the half-hearted health claims shouldn't keep you from consuming tomatoes and tomato products, however. Besides being rich in lycopene, tomatoes are a good source of lutein, which research has associated with a reduced risk of macular degeneration, the leading cause of vision loss and blindness in people age 65 and older. A single medium-sized tomato also contains half your daily value of vitamin C.

Just watch out for processed tomato products that may add a lot of salt and sugar: A typical 15-ounce can of tomato sauce (supposedly seven quarter-cup servings), for example, contains a total of 1,820 milligrams of sodium, 77% of your daily value. Either cook up fresh tomatoes or seek out the no-salt-added canned varieties.

To learn more: FDA Letter of Partial Denial, <www.cfsan.fda.gov/~dms/qhclyco2.html%20>. American Cancer Society: Food and Fitness, <www. cancer.org/docroot/PED/ped_3.asp?sitearea=PED>.

Lose Belly Fat to Lower Colon Cancer Risk

Need another reason to lose that "spare tire"? A large European study suggests that adults who carry much of their fat around the middle may be at increased risk for colon cancer.

The findings come from the EPIC study (European Prospective Investigation into Cancer and Nutrition), a large ongoing study of nutrition and cancer risk among European adults. Researchers found that among 368,277 adults from nine European countries, men and women with more abdominal fat—carrying the proverbial "spare tire"—were more likely to develop colon cancer than those who were trimmer around the middle.

The researchers examined data on men and women who had their weight and body measurements taken and who completed questionnaires on diet, exercise and other lifestyle factors at the start of the study. Over the next six years, men with the largest waist-to-hip ratio were 51% more likely than their slimmer counterparts to be diagnosed with colon cancer; women with the most belly fat had a 52% higher risk than those women with the smallest waist-to-hip ratio. Subjects simply with the largest waistlines also had a higher risk than the slimmest groups (39% for men and 48% for women).

The study, published in the *Journal of the National Cancer Institute*, suggests that abdominal fat holds particular weight when it comes to colon-cancer risk. Tobias Pischon, MD, MPH, a researcher at the German Institute of Human Nutrition in Potsdam-Rehbruecke and the lead author of the study, said the study points to the importance of preventing abdominal obesity in particular, as that type of fat is more "metabolically active." Abdominal fat may raise colon-cancer risk by increasing the levels of certain hormones that affect cell growth, including cancer cells.

The researchers found that body weight and body-mass index (BMI) were related to colon-cancer risk in men but not in women. In contrast, abdominal fat was equally strongly related to colon-cancer risk in both men and women. One explanation, according to Pischon's team, may be the difference between the way men and women carry extra weight. When a man has a high BMI, it's typically because of fat around the middle. But women tend to carry their fat around the hips and thighs, so waist size may be a more accurate predictor of colon cancer risk than overall BMI, particularly for women, according to Pischon.

"Our study shows that it's more important to keep an eye on the waist circumference, especially in women," he said.

> **TO LEARN MORE:** *Journal of the National Cancer Institute*, July 5, 2006; abstract at <jncicancerspectrum.oxfordjournals.org/cgi/content/abstract/jnci;98/13/920>.

Keep the Pounds Off to Reduce Breast Cancer Risk

Just in case you needed one more good reason to shed those extra pounds, a new study links obesity and breast cancer risk. Unlike genetics or family history, researchers point out, weight is at least a risk factor women can do something about.

The study by American Cancer Society researchers drew on data from more than 44,000 postmenopausal women who participated in the ACS Cancer Prevention Study II Nutrition Cohort. The women were not taking hormone-replacement therapy. The study focused on 1,200 women with invasive breast cancers.

Compared with women who had gained only 20 pounds or less after age 18, those in the study who had gained 60 pounds or more as adults had elevated risk for every tumor type, stage and grade. The heavier women were nearly twice as likely to have ductal type tumors, and their risk of cancer that spread beyond the breast was triple that of their slimmer counterparts.

Breast cancer risk is linked to increased levels of estrogen, which fat tissue produces.

Some have suggested a link between obesity and risk of breast cancer might be because tumors are harder to find—by manual exam or mammography—in heavier women. But the cancer-society researchers said it is more likely that the increased fat tissue raises the level of estrogen circulating in the body, thereby increasing the risk for estrogen-positive tumors.

"Our findings are especially relevant to current medical practice and public health issues given the recent decline in postmenopausal hormone use and the increasing prevalence of overweight and obesity in the United States and other Westernized countries," noted lead author Heather Spencer Feigelson, PhD, MPH.

Breast cancer is the second leading cause of death from cancer among US women, after lung cancer. More than 200,000 cases are diagnosed each year, and some 40,000 women die annually from the disease.

"Adult weight gain is one of the few well-established risk factors for breast cancer that is modifiable," Feigelson points out. "These data further illustrate the relation between adult weight gain and breast cancer and the importance of maintaining a healthy body weight throughout adulthood."

To learn more: *Cancer*, July 1, 2006; abstract at <www3.interscience.wiley.com/cgi-bin/abstract/ 112635067>.

Vitamin D May Protect Against Breast Cancer

Two studies presented at the annual meeting of the American Association for Cancer Research (AACR) suggest a potentially promising line of investigation for reducing the risk of breast cancer. Both appear to link higher levels of vitamin D with lower incidence of breast cancer.

Such a connection had been suspected, because women who live at lower, sunnier latitudes have lower rates of breast cancer than those at more northern latitudes. That holds true even when diet and other factors are taken into account.

One presentation at the conference was an analysis of pooled data from two studies on a total of 1,760 women. The women were divided into five groups ("quintiles") based on their blood levels of vitamin D. The researchers, from the University of California at San Diego, found what's called a "dose-response" relationship between vitamin D levels and breast-cancer risk: The risk dropped steadily with each quintile of higher vitamin D. Statistical analysis of the data indicated that women with very high levels of vitamin D would have a 50% lower risk than those with the lowest level.

That extremely high level, however, would actually require a vitamin D intake of 2,700 International Units (IU) daily—above the National Academy of Sciences' safe upper limit of 2,400 IU daily. The average amount of vitamin D that US women get daily is only 320 IU.

Lead researcher Cedric Garland, PhD, said the results suggest that "consideration should be given to revising the upper limit and the adequate intake (200-800 IU/day), and to greater fortification of food with vitamin D3," which is more potent than the more commonly found D2 form of the vitamin. He added, "We think it is time to take action based on the dose-response relationship seen in these studies."

In a second presentation at the AACR meeting, Julia A. Knight, PhD, of Mount Sinai Hospital in Toronto reported on an analysis of data on 576 women with breast cancer and 813 age-matched women without the disease. That study showed associations between reduced breast-cancer risk and sources of vitamin D in women's diets (milk, cod liver oil) and lifestyles (outdoor work or other outdoor activity where sunlight can trigger the body's natural ability to make vitamin D). Exposure to vitamin D early in life, especially around adolescence when the breasts are developing, was most strongly linked to a preventive benefit.

While cautioning that further investigation is needed, Knight added, "It's becoming clearer now that vitamin D is more important than people used to think."

To learn more: American Association for Cancer Research <www.aacr.org>.

Protecting Your Joints and Bones

Glucosamine & Chondroitin Don't Help Most with Osteoarthritis

The largest study yet of glucosamine and chondroitin, supplements popularly thought to fight arthritis pain, has found no clear benefit for most patients. Results of the Glucosamine/Chrondroitin Arthritis Intervention Trial (GAIT), funded by the National Institutes of Health (NIH), were reported at the annual scientific meeting of the American College of Rheumatology.

A small subgroup, about 20% of the study subjects with moderate or severe osteoarthritis, did see a statistically significant benefit from the supplements. And the annual meeting also heard results of a smaller, industry-funded European study of a prescription form of glucosamine, not available in the US, which found it more effective against osteoarthritis pain than acetaminophen.

The GAIT study was a randomized, double-blind trial involving 1,538 patients at 16 US academic medical centers. Participants were allowed to take Tylenol (acetaminophen) except within 24 hours of study visits. They were assigned to one of five treatment groups: glucosamine hydrochloride, chondroitin sulfate, a glucosamine-chondroitin combination, the painkiller Celebrex or a placebo.

Although Celebrex worked, the supplements failed to fight pain for a majority of subjects. Neither supplement nor the combination showed significantly better results than the placebo for the main study group in the goal of achieving a 20% reduction in knee pain after 24 weeks.

"For the study as a whole, the supplements were not shown to be effective," said co-author Daniel O. Clegg, MD, chief of rheumatology at the University of Utah School of Medicine. "However, an exploratory analysis

Q My son-in-law is troubled with arthritis in his hands. My daughter read "somewhere" that eating cherries might alleviate the problem. Is there any evidence that eating cherries or drinking cherry juice will help against arthritis?

A Sour cherries in particular have long been used in folk medicine as a remedy for inflammation. Today, scientists are exploring the possible benefits of antioxidants in cherries and other fruits. Cherries contain antioxidants, including kaempferol and quercetin, which may have anti-inflammatory effects. Most red-colored fruits also contain cyanidin, an antioxidant that helps give them their color. A 2005 Chinese study of the effects of cyanidin from cherries on inflammation in rats concluded that it "could be one of the potential candidates for the alleviation of arthritis."

But the findings to date are a long way from a prescription for guzzling cherry juice or gobbling cherries to fight arthritis. In fact, last year the US Food and Drug Administration (FDA) sent warning letters to 29 cherry marketers to stop making "unproven claims" for the fruit's medicinal qualities—including cancer, heart disease, gout, diabetes and arthritis.

The Arthritis Foundation "does not see any harm in eating cherries for antioxidant protection, but does not believe there is enough proven clinical evidence to suggest that eating cherries is beneficial for reducing the pain and inflammation associated with arthritis."

suggested that the combination of glucosamine and chondroitin sulfate might be effective in osteoarthritis patients who had moderate to severe knee pain. Given the results of this study, patients might want to discuss treatment options with their physicians."

In the subgroup with moderate-to-severe pain, 79.2% taking the glucosamine-chondroitin combination experienced pain relief, compared with 69.4% on Celebrex and 54.3% on a placebo.

The other study, a multicenter Spanish trial, compared a different formulation, glucosamine sulfate, against acetaminophen and a placebo in 318 patients. The researchers concluded that "a prescription of oral glucosamine sulfate at a dose of 1.5 grams per day should be the preferred medication for osteoarthritis patients."

Dr. Clegg believes the apparent difference from his GAIT results was due not to the glucosamine formulation but to higher baseline pain levels in the European test.

To learn more: American College of Rheumatology
<www.rheumatology.org/press/ 2005/clegg.asp>. Arthritis Foundation
<www. arthritis.org/research/acr_meeting/GAITStatement_final_11_10_05.pdf>.

Vitamin D Drives Bone Health–and You May Not Be Getting Enough

Evidence continues to mount of the important role vitamin D plays in maintaining healthy bones. A new Icelandic study has concluded, in fact, that if you aren't getting enough vitamin D, it may not matter how much calcium you're consuming.

The researchers studied 944 adults, ages 30 to 85, using food questionnaires and tests for blood levels of vitamin D, calcium and serum intact parathyroid hormone (PTH). A protein hormone secreted by the parathyroid gland, PTH is the most important regulator of body calcium and phosphorus and is a key indicator of bone health. The study found that higher levels of vitamin D were more closely associated than high calcium levels with normal PTH.

That means, the scientists suggested in the *Journal of the American Medical Association*, you may not need more than 800 International Units (IU) daily of calcium—as long as you're getting plenty of vitamin D.

Even Moderate Exercise Staves Off Arthritis Decline

Even a little bit of exercise can help prevent disability from arthritis, according to a new Northwestern University study. Researchers followed 3,554 adults ages 53-63 with osteoarthritis, the most common form of the ailment, taking part in the Health and Retirement Study. They divided participants into three groups based on their reported leisure activities at the study's start: inactive, "insufficiently active" and those getting the recommended amount of exercise for adults–at least 30 minutes of moderate activity or 20 minutes of vigorous exercise on most days of the week.

Over a two-year span, the most active group proved 41% less likely to show functional decline–problems with daily tasks such as walking, climbing stairs and doing basic chores–than the inactive group. But the risk reduction was almost as great–38%–for the arthritis patients in the middle, "insufficiently active" group.

"Given the high prevalence of arthritis," concluded lead author Joe Feinglass, PhD, "even modest increases in rates of lifestyle physical activity among older adults could make a substantial contribution to disability-free life expectancy."

To learn more: *Arthritis Care & Research*, Dec. 7, 2005; free abstract at <www3.interscience.wiley.com/cgi-bin/abstract/ 112193115/ABSTRACT>.

Moreover, vitamin D can even make up for a shortfall in calcium, although the reverse is not true. "Our results suggest that vitamin D sufficiency can ensure ideal serum PTH values even when the calcium intake level is less than 800 milligrams/day," wrote lead author Laufey Steingrimsdotter, PhD, of the Public Health Institute of Iceland, "while high calcium intake (greater than 1,200 milligrams/day) is not sufficient to maintain ideal serum PTH, as long as vitamin D status is insufficient."

How much vitamin D do you need? Because it's difficult to get enough vitamin D from dietary sources alone, the researchers recommended vitamin D supplements of approximately 500 IU daily. In northern climes such as Iceland as well as the northern US and Canada, you must also compensate for the lack of sunshine—which stimulates the body's natural vitamin D production—in winter. During winter months, the study found approximately 700 IU daily of vitamin D was required to maintain adequate levels for sufficient PTH.

To learn more: *Journal of the American Medical Association*, Nov. 9, 2005. Free abstract at
<jama. ama-assn.org/cgi/content/abstract/294/18/2336>

New Twist on Back Pain Treatment– Yoga

If you suffer chronic back pain, a new study suggests giving yoga class a try. Researchers at the Group Health Cooperative in Seattle compared three types of treatment among 101 back patients: a self-help book, aerobic exercise and a gentle form of yoga called viniyoga. The back-pain sufferers were randomly assigned to one of the three treatment groups, and were interviewed after six and 12 weeks, plus 14 weeks after treatment ended. At 12 weeks, 78% of the yoga group had experienced at least a two-point improvement on the Roland Disability Scale, compared to 63% in the aerobics group and 47% in the book group. Although "symptom bothersomeness" was rated about the same among all treatments at the conclusion, the yoga group scored significantly better 14 weeks later; also, only 21% required pain medication at that point, compared to 50% in the aerobics group and 59% in the self-help book group.

"Yoga may be beneficial for back pain because it involves physical movement, but it may also exert benefits through its effects on mental focus," the researchers commented.

To learn more: *Annals of Internal Medicine*, Dec. 20, 2005. Free abstract at
<www.annals.org/cgi/content/full/ 143/12/849>.

Calcium, Vitamin D and Bone Health: Now What Should You Do?

The ink was hardly dry on the controversial news about low-fat diets from the Women's Health Initiative when a second arm of the study reported more results that seemed to contradict conventional medical wisdom: In a seven-year trial of 36,282 postmenopausal women, researchers found no significant benefit from calcium and vitamin D supplementation in preventing hip fractures.

Based on previous studies, calcium supplements have long been a key weapon in the battle against osteoporosis, a loss of bone density that's especially common in women after menopause. Americans spend nearly a billion dollars annually on calcium supplements, the biggest seller in the dietary-supplement industry. Vitamin D, a key partner in this equation, has been shown to promote the body's absorption of calcium.

But the new findings from the National Heart, Lung and Blood Institute's Women's Health Initiative (WHI), published in the *New England Journal of Medicine,* triggered a wave of headlines suggesting that everything scientists thought they knew about calcium, vitamin D and bone health was wrong. Not only did the women in the supplement group not experience significantly fewer fractures of the hip or other bones than those in the control group—they also saw a 17% increase in the risk of kidney stones. The message seemed clear: Throw away your calcium and vitamin D pills.

Bess Dawson-Hughes, MD, director of the Bone Metabolism Laboratory at Tufts' Jean Mayer USDA Human Nutrition Research Center on Aging, thinks that's a dangerous—and inaccurate—message. "It's really unfortunate how this has been interpreted," she says. "A lot of people may be harmed by this."

For most people age 50 and up, men as well as women, Dr. Dawson-Hughes hasn't changed her recommendations at all in the wake of the WHI results: Follow the National Academies' guidelines of 1,200 milligrams of calcium daily, plus aim for 800-1,000 international units (IU) of vitamin D daily. That vitamin D intake is more than the current Academies' guidelines of 400 IU for ages 61-70 and 600 IU for ages 71 and up, but those 1997 numbers may be reconsidered in light of other recent research.

"Most people should not stop their calcium and vitamin D supplementation," says Dr. Dawson-Hughes. "It remains very important for menopausal women and others to meet the evidence-based calcium and vitamin D requirements. This study doesn't do anything to undermine that recommendation, and in fact indirectly supports it."

The only people who should make a change based on the WHI findings, she adds, are the rare few getting much more calcium than recommended.

In light of the increased risk of kidney stones at high calcium levels, it's probably smart to cut back to 1,200 milligrams.

Even WHI director Elizabeth G. Nabel, MD, agrees the new findings don't mean most older woman should stop taking supplements. "The overall results suggest that women, particularly those over 60, should consider taking calcium and vitamin D for bone health," she said in a statement. And study lead author Rebecca D. Jackson, MD, of Ohio State University, echoed that advice: "We still do believe… that maintaining an adequate calcium intake will lay the foundation for bone health."

To understand why many experts aren't jumping on the calcium-bashing media bandwagon over the WHI report, it helps to read the study's fine print. Roughly half the subjects, who ranged in age from 50-79, were assigned to take 1,000 milligrams of calcium and 400 IU of vitamin D supplements daily; the other half were placed in a placebo group. But the researchers allowed the women in both groups to take up to 1,000 milligrams of calcium and up to 600 IU of vitamin D daily on top of whatever they were (or were not) getting in the clinical trial. About a third of the placebo group took their own supplements during the study, and as a result many had adequate calcium-intake levels anyway. Half the women also continued on hormone therapy.

These factors, critics note, would tend to flatten any differences between the groups. In effect, the study actually compared women taking an average 2,150 milligrams of calcium daily with those taking an average 1,150 milligrams—very nearly the recommended intake of 1,200 milligrams.

The test group did see a tiny benefit in hip-bone density and a 12% reduction in fracture rate—neither difference deemed statistically significant. Overall, both groups experienced less than half the expected rate of fractures, leading the authors to concede that the study was "underpowered" to detect benefits from supplementation.

The level of vitamin D tested—400 IU—was also only half what most experts now recommend, Dr. Dawson-Hughes points out. Though test subjects saw a small increase in blood levels of vitamin D, they reached only two-thirds the level needed to reduce fracture rates, according to recent studies. The need for this higher level of vitamin D was not apparent when the study was designed.

Finally, despite the negative headlines, some subsets in the study did see significant benefits. Those age 60 and older—the population most in danger of debilitating fractures—experienced a 21% decrease in risk. The women who consistently followed the full supplement regimen saw a 29% risk reduction. (By the study's end, only 59% of the participants were taking as many supplements as the trial required.) And those who were not taking their own supplements during the study cut their hip fracture risk by 30%.

Bone Testing Missing Those Most at Risk

Osteoporosis screening can lead to drug or hormone treatment that reduces the risk of debilitating fractures. But the women who could most benefit from such screening are the least likely to get it, according to a new study. Researchers at the Medical College of Wisconsin in Milwaukee found that as women age–and become at greater risk for osteoporosis–they are less likely to be screened for the bone-thinning condition. In an analysis of 44,000 women, the investigators found that 27% of those age 66 to 70 got screened in a three-year period. But less than 10% of the oldest women, ages 80 to 90, were screened.

The US Preventive Services Task Force recommends bone-density testing for osteoporosis for all women 65 and older. Medicare, which began covering the cost of screening in 1999, the first year analyzed in the study, will pay for the test every two years.

The risk of osteoporosis jumps with age, afflicting less than 20% of women ages 65 to 74 but more than 50% of women over age 85. According to lead author Joan M. Neuner, MD, MPH, 40% of white women age 50 and older will suffer an osteoporosis-related fracture of the hip, wrist or spine at some point in their life-time. More than half of those with hip fractures never fully recover, and 20% will end up in a nursing home.

TO LEARN MORE: *Journal of the American Geriatrics Society*, March 2006; free abstract at <www.blackwellpublishing.com/jgs>. National Osteoporosis Foundation, 1232 22nd St. NW, Washington, DC 20037, (202) 223-2226, <www.nof.org>.

"Many statisticians don't think one should look at these subsets," Dr. Dawson-Hughes says, "but when there's a biologically plausible reason to do so, when it fits with prior evidence, it makes sense."

Though the study focused on women, Dr. Dawson-Hughes adds that men also need to be concerned about bone health. Anyone over age 50 should make sure to get enough calcium and vitamin D; weight-bearing exercises can also help build strong bones. Surveys have shown that most American women get only about half the recommended 1,200 milligrams of calcium daily. Without a radical dietary change—hard to sustain over the long term, Dr. Dawson-Hughes notes—that probably means taking calcium supplements. And despite the increasing number of fortified foods, it's hard to get enough vitamin D from diet alone; a supplement and 15 minutes of safe sun exposure can help.

To learn more: *New England Journal of Medicine*, Feb. 16, 2006; free abstract online at <content.nejm.org/ cgi/content/abstract/354/7/669>.
National Osteoporosis Foundation, 1232 22nd St. NW, Washington, DC 20037, (202) 223-2226, <www.nof.org>.
Strong Women, Strong Bones by Miriam E. Nelson, PhD, with Sarah Wernick, PhD (Perigee, $14.95, available at <www.tuftsbooks.com>).

Keeping Your Brain Sharp as You Age

Protecting Your Heart May Also Benefit Your Brain

Heart-healthy habits such as staying physically active and controlling your blood pressure may also protect your brain. A blue-ribbon panel of the National Institutes of Health (NIH) Cognitive and Emotional Health Project, which reviewed 96 studies on factors affecting the brain, found significant parallels between cardiovascular health and both cognitive and emotional health in people over 65.

"A large variety of risk factors were consistently identified with cognitive outcomes, particularly those previously associated with increased risk of cardiovascular disease," the report, published in *Alzheimer's & Dementia: The Journal of the Alzheimer's Association*, concluded. "There was considerable overlap between risk factors for cognitive and emotional outcomes."

The strongest link across studies was between high blood pressure and cognitive decline, according to committee chair Hugh Hendrie, MB, ChB, DSc, professor of psychiatry at Indiana University School of Medicine. Controlling hypertension may be one of the most important interventions not only for preventing cardiovascular trouble, the panel noted, but also for fighting cognitive decline.

Across the studies, other factors consistently associated with cognitive decline, in addition to age, were: diabetes, stroke or transient ischemic attacks, infarcts or white matter lesions on brain imaging, low mood scores and higher body mass index (BMI).

Physical activity seemed to be protective against cognitive decline, much as it helps ward off heart disease. If confirmed, this association "would be of great public health importance because physical activity is relatively inexpensive, has few negative consequences, and is accessible to most elders," the report noted.

The NIH committee looked at long-term studies with at least 500 participants, predominantly involving subjects age 65 and older.

"Many of the factors that can put our brain health at risk are things we can modify and control," said William Thies, PhD, vice president for medical and scientific affairs of the Alzheimer's Association. "This points to the possibility that healthier living can significantly contribute to reducing the numbers of sick and mentally declining older people, and reduce healthcare costs."

To learn more: Alzheimer's & Dementia: *The Journal of the Alzheimer's Association*, Jan. 2006; free abstract at <www.alzheimersanddementia.com>. Alzheimer's Association <www.alz.org/News/06Q1/022106.asp>. National Institute on Aging <www.nia.nih.gov/alzheimers>.

6 Keys to Heart Health Also Predict Dementia Risk

If you're already changing your lifestyle to fight heart disease, there's good news: You may be helping to prevent Alzheimer's disease and other forms of dementia at the same time. New research from the Karolinska Institute in Sweden suggests that six factors in middle age are associated with the risk of dementia later in life. The lifestyle-related risk predictors were the same as those previously linked to heart disease and stroke—high blood pressure, high cholesterol levels, obesity and lack of exercise—along with low educational attainment and advancing age.

In the study, published in the British journal *The Lancet Neurology*, researchers analyzed data on 1,409 individuals who were assessed for signs of dementia at about age 50 and again 20 years later. Only 4% of this group actually developed dementia, but these subjects had the highest risk score on the factors being studied. Individuals were scored according to how they fit the six factors; risk of dementia rose from 1% for those with the lowest scores to 16.4% in the highest-scoring group.

It's significant that these risk factors for dementia are the same as those for cardiovascular disease, noted lead researcher Miia Kivipelto, MD. The findings, she added, open new avenues for prevention: "This approach highlights the role of vascular factors in the development of dementia and could help to identify individuals who might benefit from intensive lifestyle consultations and pharmacological interventions."

Dr. Kivipelto and her colleagues also cautioned, "The dementia risk score is a novel approach for the prediction of dementia risk, but should be validated and further improved to increase its predictive value."

To learn more: *The Lancet Neurology,* Sept. 2006; abstract at <www.thelancet.com/journals/ laneur/article/ PIIS1474442206705373/abstract>.

Don't Put Off Exercise–Put Off Alzheimer's Instead

Frequent exercise seems to delay the onset of Alzheimer's disease and other forms of dementia, according to a new study published in the *Annals of Internal Medicine.* The findings add to the mounting evidence that keeping active can help keep your mind sharp as you age.

Researchers at Group Health Cooperative in Seattle followed 1,740 adults age 65 and older with normal mental function. The study asked participants how many days a week they got at least 15 minutes of physical activity; no effort was made to measure how hard they exercised, just how often. Over an average 6.2-year span, 107 participants were diagnosed with Alzheimer's, 51 developed other forms of dementia, and 1,158 remained free of dementia. (The rest either dropped out of the study or died.) Of those who didn't develop dementia, 77% exercised three or more times weekly, compared to 67% of those who did get dementia.

When the scientists looked at the group that exercised at least three times weekly, they found a 32% less risk of dementia than infrequent or non-exercisers. Those who were frailest at the start of the study actually benefited the most.

The study is the "first to report an interaction between level of physical function and physical activity and dementia risk," noted an accompanying editorial by Laura Podewils, PhD, of the Centers for Disease Control, and Eliseo Guallar, MD, DrPH, of Johns Hopkins.

Exercise may help delay dementia by improving the blood flow in the brain, especially to areas involved in memory, suggested lead author Eric B. Larson, MD. But Dr. Larson cautioned that this study does not prove a cause-and-effect relationship between exercise and dementia risk.

The results do jibe with an earlier Johns Hopkins study that found participants in the widest variety of activities were significantly less likely to develop dementia. Previous studies have also found that exercise can help combat depression in the elderly: A 2003 study by some of the same Seattle-based researchers as this latest work found exercise effective against depression in patients already suffering from Alzheimer's. And research by Nalin A. Singh, FRACP, and Maria A. Fiatarone Singh, MD, a visiting scientist at Tufts' Jean Mayer USDA Human Nutrition Research Center on Aging, has shown that high-intensity weight-lifting exercise is as effective (about 60% improvement in symptoms) as antidepressant medications in depressed elderly patients.

So there's definitely a connection between your head and the activity level in the rest of your body. If these latest findings are confirmed, according to Dr. Larson, exercise could be an important weapon against "one of the most feared illnesses of aging. ... Physicians and health-promotion programs might find this information valuable as our society works to find truly effective ways to promote physical activity for all its well-known health benefits."

To learn more: *Annals of Internal Medicine*, Jan. 17, 2006; online at <www.annals.org/cgi/content/full/144/2/73>. Alzheimer's Disease Education & Referral Center <www.alzheimers.org>.

Midlife Exercise May Reduce Later Dementia Risk

If you're a middle-aged couch potato, here's yet another reason to get off your duff: Regular exercise now may help prevent dementia and Alzheimer's disease later. Researchers at the Aging Research Center of the Karolinska Institute in Sweden have found that exercising at least twice weekly in midlife reduces the risk of dementia by more than 50% and the risk of Alzheimer's disease by more than 60%.

According to lead author Miia Kivipelto, MD, PhD, this is the first study to show a long-term relationship between physical activity and dementia later in life.

The population-based cohort study, published in The Lancet Neurology, surveyed and examined 1,449 participants at midlife and again an average of 21 years later, at ages 65-79. At the follow-up examination, 117 participants showed evidence of dementia and 76 had been diagnosed with Alzheimer's disease. Those who had exercised at least twice a week at the initial, midlife examination—781 of the participants—had a greatly reduced risk for dementia and Alzheimer's disease, even after adjusting for other lifestyle and health factors.

The greatest benefit from midlife exercise was seen in people with a genetic susceptibility to dementia and Alzheimer's, those having a gene labeled apoE4.

No connection was found between the level of exercise and the degree of risk reduction. Any physical activity vigorous enough to cause sweating and strained breathing seemed to qualify; walking and cycling were the most common forms of activity among participants.

The researchers couldn't explain how physical activity reduces the risk of dementia and Alzheimer's. They theorized, however, that exercise might directly affect the brain's messaging system, as well as improving blood flow to the brain.

To learn more: *The Lancet Neurology*, November 2005. Free abstract online at <www.sciencedirect.com/science/journal/ 14744422>.
Alzheimer's Disease Education & Referral Center <www.alzheimers.org>.

Mediterranean-Style Diet Pattern Could Reduce Risk of Alzheimer's Disease

Scientists are taking a closer look at the connections between what you eat and your risk of Alzheimer's disease and cognitive decline. In a recently published Columbia University study, researchers found an association between reduced Alzheimer's risk and a dietary pattern similar to the so-called "Mediterranean diet." And several related dietary factors were in the spotlight at a special International Academy of Nutrition and Aging's (IANA) conference on nutrition, Alzheimer's disease and cognitive decline.

The new study, published in *Annals of Neurology*, followed 2,258 elderly northern Manhattanites over an average of four years. Every 18 months, they were evaluated with a dozen neuropsychological tests and given a food questionnaire. Over the span of the study, 262 participants were diagnosed as developing Alzheimer's disease.

Researchers used a nine-point scale to measure subjects' adherence to elements of a Mediterranean-style diet. Although there's no single true "Mediterranean diet"—people in Tunisia eat differently from those in, say, Greece—certain common components of the region's diet have previously been linked to a reduced risk of cardiovascular disease. In the Columbia study, scientists looked for:
- High intake of vegetables, legumes, fruits, fish and cereals
- High intake of unsaturated fatty acids but low intake of saturated lipids
- Low intake of dairy products, meat and poultry
- Mild to moderate alcohol consumption

Even after adjusting for demographics and known risk factors, adherence to the Mediterranean-style dietary pattern remained the main predictor of Alzheimer's risk. Each additional unit of adherence to the diet was associated with a 9-10% reduced risk. The one-third of the subjects who followed the diet most closely had a 39-40% lower risk of Alzheimer's than the group with the lowest adherence.

Presentations at the special IANA symposium in Chicago mirrored many of the nutritional elements in the study. Co-sponsored by Rush University's Institute for Healthy Aging, the conference looked at the possible protective benefits of B vitamins and polyphenols—both found in fruits and vegetables—as well as polyunsaturated fatty acids, especially the omega-3s found in certain fish.

But another possible lesson of the Columbia research is that it's not just individual nutrients that may offer protection from cognitive decline—it's the whole dietary pattern. Although mild to moderate alcohol intake and high vegetable consumption were each associated with decreased risk, after further adjustment for other factors, no individual component proved a significant risk predictor. According to lead researcher Nikolaos Scarmeas, MD, "An overall dietary pattern is likely to have a greater effect on human health than a single nutrient."

Mediterranean-style diets, Dr. Scarmeas speculated, may be effective against Alzheimer's by combating inflammation and oxidative stress. Also, a blue-ribbon National Institutes of Health panel recently found significant parallels between cardiovascular health and cognitive health in people over 65. So the Mediterranean diet patterns' demonstrated cardiovascular benefits may translate into protection for the brain.

To learn more: *Annals of Neurology*, published online in advance of print <www3.interscience.wiley.com/cgi-bin/abstract/112593516/ABSTRACT>.

B Vitamins and Folate Fall Short on Brain Benefits

While folate and B vitamins are effective at lowering levels of an amino acid, homocysteine, that's been linked to heart disease and dementia, they don't necessarily combat those health problems. Three large studies testing folate and B vitamins against heart disease recently reported negative results. Now a trial of the nutrients' impact on cognitive function has found the folate and B vitamins combination no more effective than a placebo.

Researchers at the University of Otago in New Zealand had theorized that by lowering homocysteine levels, the folate and B vitamins would improve mental performance. The nutrients did succeed in significantly dropping homocysteine levels. But despite their reduced levels of the suspect amino acid, healthy, highly functioning older adults taking the vitamins did no better than a similar control group on a battery of eight cognitive tests. The findings were published in the *New England Journal of Medicine*.

The study randomly split 276 participants, all age 65 or older and with elevated homocysteine levels, into two groups. One group took a daily supplement of 1,000 micrograms of folate, 500 micrograms of B-12 and 10 milligrams of B-6; the other half got a look-alike dummy pill. After two years, scores on the mental tests failed to turn up any statistically significant differences between the vitamin and placebo groups.

The study was a double-blind, placebo-controlled, randomized clinical trial—considered the "gold standard" for scientific research. But the relatively small number of subjects and short duration of the trial led some experts to be cautious about drawing too sweeping a conclusion from the results. In an accompanying editorial in the same journal issue, Robert Clarke, MD, of the University of Oxford in England—a proponent of the benefits of lowering homocysteine—wrote that the study "lacked the statistical power to refute the homocysteine hypothesis of dementia."

The study's lead author, C. Murray Skeaff, PhD, pointed out, "Our study was designed to examine the effect of homocysteine on cognitive performance; our trial was not designed to examine the effect of homocysteine-lowering on dementia, for which studies of long duration are required. If dementia is at the extreme of the continuum of cognitive decline, then according to the 'homocysteine hypothesis' we might have expected better cognitive performance in the vitamins group. This did not happen."

Bill Thies, PhD, Alzheimer's Association vice president, medical and scientific relations, commented, "We'd love to have something that is simple and reproducible and cheap and effective that protect against cognitive decline and dementia," but he said the possibility that vitamin supplements are such a "magic bullet" remains an open question.

More definitive word could come from the B-Vitamin Treatment Trialists' Collaboration, which has gathered up to seven years of data from 12 large clinical trials to explore the effect of B vitamins on cardiovascular function. Dr. Clarke suggested that the same data could also be used to further test possible cognitive benefits.

To learn more: *New England Journal of Medicine*, June 29, 2006; abstract at <content.nejm.org/cgi/content/short/354/26/2764>. Alzheimer's Association <www.alz.org>.

A Glass of Juice Every Other Day May Keep Alzheimer's Away

That morning glass of juice may do more than just perk you up at breakfast time. A new study suggests that a glass of fruit or vegetable juice at least every other day may help fend off Alzheimer's disease.

Researchers found that those who drank at least three glasses of fruit or vegetable juice per week were 76% less likely to develop the disease compared with those who averaged less than one glass per week. Even those who drank only one or two servings weekly had some protection (16%) compared with those who consumed less juice, reported lead author Qi Dai, MD, PhD, assistant professor of medicine at the Vanderbilt School of Medicine.

"These findings are new and suggest that fruit and vegetable juices may play an important role in delaying the onset of Alzheimer's disease," Dr. Dai and colleagues wrote in *The American Journal of Medicine*.

In the study, nearly 2,000 dementia-free Japanese-Americans living in the Seattle area—roughly half men, half women, with an average age of nearly 72—completed a food frequency questionnaire and underwent clinical evaluation. They were re-evaluated every two years for the next nine years.

The study was part of the Kame Project, a cross-national study with collaborators in Hawaii and Japan examining age-related impairment to memory and cognitive function. Alzheimer's is relatively uncommon in Japan, but its prevalence has been rising among Japanese-Americans, suggesting environmental and lifestyle factors may be at work, the investigators said.

Despite the initial promise of antioxidant vitamins for preventing Alzheimer's disease, recent study results have been disappointing, researchers noted, causing them to focus instead on polyphenol-rich fruit and vegetable juices. Although the current study did not identify the kinds of juices participants consumed, previous studies have shown that apple, grape and citrus fruit juices are high in polyphenols, which are particularly rich in the skin and peel of fruits and vegetables.

Even though the initial results were promising, Dr. Dai cautioned that the general public should not jump the gun regarding the value of juice as a preventive measure for Alzheimer's disease. "A few years ago, hormone replacement therapy, NSAIDs (nonsteroidal anti-inflammatory drugs) and antioxidant vitamins showed promise, but recent clinical trials indicate that they do not," he said. "More study, I think, is needed."

The researchers said future studies will attempt to confirm these results by measuring blood levels of polyphenols in juice drinkers and examining the relation between these levels and Alzheimer's risk.

To learn more: *The American Journal of Medicine*, September 2006, abstract at <www.amjmed.com/article/ PIIS0002934306006772/abstract>.

The Facts on Fish

For Most, Health Benefits Outweigh Risks of Eating Fish

Is concern over mercury in fish causing you to cut back on consuming seafood? If so, you could be missing out on the healthy effects of fish on everything from your cardiovascular system to your brain.

In 2004, the US Food and Drug Administration (FDA) and Environmental Protection Agency (EPA) jointly issued a warning about levels of mercury—in the form of a compound, methylmercury—in certain fish species. Like a similar advisory in 2001, the advice to avoid high-mercury species and limit total fish intake was chiefly aimed at women of child-bearing age. But experts worry that the government warnings scared Americans of all genders and ages away from seafood.

"If you are not pregnant and are not going to become pregnant, you shouldn't even be thinking about mercury in fish," says Josh Cohen, PhD, of the research staff at the Tufts New England Medical Center in the Institute for Clinical Research and Health Policy Studies. Cohen, previously affiliated with the Harvard School of Public Health, is the lead author of a three-year study by that school's Center for Risk Analysis published recently in the *American Journal of Preventive Medicine*, analyzing the pros and cons of fish consumption.

Government warnings about mercury in fish may do more harm than good to public health, the study concludes. "Fish are an excellent source of omega-3 fatty acids, which may protect against coronary heart disease and stroke, and are thought to aid in the neurological development of unborn babies," Cohen says. "If that information gets lost in how the public perceives this issue, then people may inappropriately curtail fish consumption and increase their risk for adverse health outcomes."

In fact, that's exactly what another new study, from the University of Maryland's Center for Food, Nutrition and Agriculture Policy (CFNAP), says has happened. The center commissioned a poll of 1,040 adults, which found 31% of the public concerned about mercury levels in fish. While 89% of US adults say they eat fish occasionally, only 36% of adults reported eating seafood at least once a week. The US Tuna Foundation, which helped fund the new center's Web site, <www.realmercuryfacts.org>, also says tuna consumption has dropped 10% since 2004.

The CFNAP poll found widespread confusion over warnings about mercury in fish. When asked to whom the advisory applies, 45% said the elderly, 35% said pre-teens and teenagers, 29% thought it also applies to men, and 30% said all Americans should avoid high-mercury species (which less than 5% could correctly identify).

To try to get Americans back in the swim of things, the National Oceanic and Atmospheric Administration (NOAA) sponsored a three-day "Seafood and Health" conference. Bill Hogarth, PhD, director of NOAA's Fisheries Service, told participants, "The scientific evidence explored today is clear and solid: eating more fish and shellfish will lead to a healthier, smarter and longer-lived US population. While there are risks associated with everything we consume, the health benefits gained from omega-3 fatty acids in fish and shellfish far outweigh the risks from contaminants for the vast majority of the population."

Omega-3s Make a Splash

It was a similar conference, held in Seattle 20 years ago, that first cast the spotlight on the benefits of omega-3 fatty acids, found in fatty, cold-water fish such as salmon, tuna, mackerel, herring and lake trout. In the 1970s, Scandinavian researchers had found evidence of seafood's cardiovascular benefits among Greenland's Inuit population. But research on omega-3s didn't really take off until that "Seafood & Health '85" symposium.

Since then, one study after another has shown the benefits of consuming seafood rich in omega-3s. A recent Tufts study, for instance, of 229 postmenopausal women previously diagnosed with coronary artery disease found that those who consumed more fish had a slower progression of plaque buildup in their arteries. (A new Rand Health study, however, seems to have dashed hopes that omega-3s might also be effective against cancer.)

"People should eat more fish," says Alice H. Lichtenstein, DSc, director of the Cardiovascular Nutrition Laboratory at Tufts' Jean Mayer USDA Human Nutrition Research Center on Aging. "Not only do you get omega-3s, but you get the benefits of a source of protein that low in saturated fat that you don't get with meat and cheese."

The American Heart Association, whose Nutrition Committee Lichtenstein chairs, recommends that healthy adults eat fish twice a week. But the CFNAP poll found that only 17% of US adults eat fish that often.

The Rise of Mercury Worries

The 2004 seafood consumption advisory warned pregnant and nursing women, women who might become pregnant and young children to avoid certain species of fish especially prone to mercury: shark, swordfish, tilefish and king mackerel. The advisory said these at-risk individuals can safely consume up to 12 ounces weekly of species low in mercury, such as shrimp, salmon, pollock, catfish and canned light tuna, and up to six ounces weekly of fish moderate in mercury, such as canned albacore tuna.

Power plants release mercury into the air; the mercury then falls into oceans and streams, where it accumulates in fish. When the government issued its warnings, many people just heard "avoid fish because of mercury."

If all Americans cut their fish consumption by one-sixth—as pregnant women apparently did following the 2001 mercury advisory—the Harvard Center for Risk Analysis study estimates an additional 8,000 deaths annually would result from heart disease and stroke. The study also found that by skipping fish entirely, mothers-to-be are missing out on the benefits of safe seafood to their unborn children's cognitive development.

Similar research by Joseph Hibbeln, MD, of the National Institutes of Health, has shown that children whose mothers eat greater amounts of fish during pregnancy demonstrate improved performance in a number of social and functional indices. According to Dr. Hibbeln, "It appears that fish in the mother's diet may be a bigger influence on childhood learning and behavior than getting the children themselves to eat fish."

If you're still fretting about mercury, you should know about selenium, which research since 1967 has shown neutralizes the toxicity of mercury in the body—and 16 of the top 25 sources of selenium are ocean fish. Nicholas Ralston, PhD, of the Energy and Environmental Research Center at the University of North Dakota, says the high amounts of selenium in commercial ocean fish protect humans from mercury's toxic effects. Recent research, he adds, is clarifying the mystery of how, exploring the "extraordinarily high binding affinity" between selenium and mercury.

The Slippery Facts on Salmon

If the bottom line on mercury in fish is simple—don't worry unless you're pregnant or planning to be—the story on contaminants in farm-raised salmon is more complicated. In 2003, the Environmental Working Group made headlines with a report on 10 farm-raised salmon it tested for PCBs—polychlorinated biphenyls—chemicals banned in 1977 that the EPA calls "probable carcinogens." The environmental group said 70% of the salmon it tested was "contaminated with PCBs at levels that raise health concerns," an average 27 parts per billion.

Exactly what level of PCBs in fish should cause concern is controversial, though—and not even different US government agencies agree. With an eye toward recreationally caught fish, where concentrated consumption of similarly contaminated fish is a worry, the EPA says not to eat more than eight ounces a month of fish containing between 24 and 58 parts per billion of PCBs. In monitoring commercially sold fish, however, the FDA allows 2,000 parts per billion of PCBs.

Jeffery A. Foran, PhD, of the Midwest Center for Environmental Science and Public Policy in Milwaukee, argues, "The FDA tolerance for PCBs is simply 20 years out of date. It has not been revised since 1985—well before many of the critical studies on PCB cognitive impairment were conducted." The contaminants in farmed salmon come from their feed, he notes, so—whatever safety level you trust—the problem could be solved by changing the composition of the feed.

In a 2004 study published in *Science*, Foran and colleagues analyzed more than two tons of salmon from around the world. The most contaminated salmon came from farms in Europe, although North and South American farm-raised fish still had more contaminants than wild salmon. After conducting the study, Foran says, his family switched to wild salmon; the study authors recommended limiting farmed salmon consumption to once a month or less.

In a response to that study, however, Jouni T. Tuomisto, MD, and a group of fellow researchers from the Finnish Centre of Excellence of Environmental Health Risk Analysis, noted that it did "not take into account any beneficial effects of eating fish.... If the main concern is the net health benefit, the decision-maker will not recommend restrictions" on farmed salmon.

Last year, Foran led another

Fishing for Omega-3s

Fish are an excellent source of two omega-3 fatty acids, EPA (eicosapentaenoic acid) and DHA (docosahexaenoic acid), essential compounds the body can't make on its own. The American Heart Association recommends eating fish twice a week (about six ounces total)—especially fatty, cold-water fish, which tend to be higher in omega-3s, as this chart based on USDA data shows:

Seafood	Omega-3 (EPA+DHA) in 3 ounces (cooked)
Farmed Atlantic Salmon	1.8 grams
Herring	1.7 grams
Wild Atlantic Salmon	1.6 grams
Blue Fin Tuna	1.3 grams
Sockeye Salmon (canned)	1.3 grams
Atlantic Mackerel	1.0 grams
Farmed Rainbow Trout	1.0 grams
Wild Rainbow Trout	0.8 grams
Sardines (canned)	0.8 grams
Swordfish	0.7 grams
Mussels	0.7 grams
Sole	0.4 grams
Tuna, white meat (canned)	0.2 grams
Wild Catfish	0.2 grams
Farmed Catfish	0.1 grams
Atlantic Cod	0.1 grams

study, published in the *Journal of Nutrition*, that again found significantly lower contaminant concentrations in wild salmon than farmed fish. Ironically, however, farmed salmon had significantly higher concentrations of healthy fatty acids. "This analysis suggests that risk of exposure to contaminants in farmed and wild salmon is partially offset by the fatty acid-associated health benefits," Foran wrote. The report cautioned, however, that young children, women of child-bearing age, pregnant women and nursing mothers might want to opt for wild salmon or other sources of omega-3s.

Tufts' Lichtenstein emphasizes the importance of balancing risks and rewards: "The risk of developing cardiovascular disease is high; it is the leading cause of death and disability in the US. The risk of adverse health effects of contaminated fish is very low, almost theoretical at this point," she says. "Of course, there is one caveat: When the knowledge base is incomplete, err on the side of caution. That would mean pregnant women and children. They should follow the latest guidelines."

"The bottom line is that people have choices," says Foran. "People can choose fish with lower contaminant concentrations such as wild salmon, and still get the omega-3 associated benefits. Women of child-bearing age, pregnant women, nursing mothers and young children have to be more careful in their choices and reduce contaminant exposure as much as possible, but they still can and should eat fish."

To learn more: *American Journal of Preventive Medicine,* November 2005; free abstract via <www. sciencedirect.com/science/journal/07493797>. Center for Food, Nutrition and Agriculture Policy <www. realmercuryfacts.org>. *Journal of Nutrition,* November 2005; free abstract at <www.nutrition.org/cgi/content/abstract/135/11/2639>. Science, Jan. 9, 2004; free abstract at <www.sciencemag.org/cgi/content/ short/303/5655/226>. US Food and Drug Administration <www.cfsan.fda.gov/seafood1.html>.

Getting a Charge Out of Fish Oil

Researchers are taking a novel approach to understanding some of the possible heart-health benefits of eating fish: Maybe fish oils help regulate the heart's electrical activity.

A recent observational study found that eating tuna or similar fish, baked or broiled—but not fried—at least once a week was associated with a slower heart rate and healthier electrical activity within the heart. Lead author Dariush Mozaffarian, MD, DrPH, of Brigham and Women's Hospital and Harvard Medical School, explains that the heart resets its electrical activity after every beat: "When the resetting of the heart's electrical activity is slowed, a person is at highest risk of sudden death." The fish eaters in the study showed a lower likelihood that the heart would take a long time to electrically reset.

The study, published in the *Journal of the American College of Cardiology*, analyzed data from 5,096 men and women, age 65 and older, participating in the Cardiovascular Heart Study. The average heart rate of those consuming the most fish was 3.5 beats per minute lower than that of the group consuming the least fish. The group with the highest fish intake had only half the risk of "prolonged QT" (a measure of the time for the heart to reset its electrical activity) seen in those eating the least fish. While heart benefits increased with greater fish consumption, significant gains were seen with just one or two meals of fish weekly.

But the jury's still out on fish oil's electrical benefits, as shown by another new study testing whether the fatty acids in fish could reduce the risk of cardiac arrhythmia in high-risk patients. The randomized, double-blind intervention study split 546 cardiac patients into two groups; over almost a year, one group got fish-oil supplements while the other got a placebo. The results, published in the *Journal of the American Medical Association,* were disappointing, with little difference between the groups. The researchers, from Wageningen University in the Netherlands, concluded, "Our findings do not indicate evidence of a strong protective effect."

Alice H. Lichtenstein, DSc, Gershoff professor at Tufts' Friedman School and chair of the American Heart Association's nutrition committee, urges caution as science continues to probe the connections between fish oils and the heart's electrical cycles. She notes, "Once again, as in the case of vitamin E, the intervention data has not supported the observational data."

To learn more: *Journal of the American College of Cardiology*, August 1, 2006. *Journal of the American Medical Association*, June 14, 2006.

Fatty Fish May Decrease Risk of Kidney Cancer

Besides the well-known heart-health benefits of eating fatty fish, regular consumption of fish such as salmon, mackerel, sardines and herring may also help prevent kidney cancer. Swedish researchers recently found that women who dined on fatty cold-water fish at least once a week had a 44% lower risk of renal-cell carcinoma, compared with women who ate no fish.

The researchers from the Karolinska Institute of Stockholm used data from the Swedish Mammography Cohort, a population-based study of more than 61,000 women ages 40 to 76 with no previous diagnosis of cancer. The women were tracked over the course of 15 years. The findings were published in the *Journal of the American Medical Association.*

US kidney and renal-pelvis cancer:
• Estimated 38,890 new cases annually
• About 12,840 deaths in 2006

Fatty cold-water fish have as much as 20 to 30 times the omega-3 fatty acids and three to five times higher levels of vitamin D than varieties such as cod, tuna and freshwater fish, or shrimp, lobster and crayfish. Lower serum vitamin D levels have been linked to the development and progression of renal-cell carcinoma, the researchers noted.

No reduction in kidney cancer incidence was seen from consumption of shellfish or freshwater fish in the study.

Lead author Alicja Wolk, DMSc, said consumers should not be scared off by the term "fatty fish," as the fish contain "good fats," and that the health benefits far outweigh any extra calories.

Previous studies have investigated a possible link between fish consumption and protection from renal-cell carcinoma. But Wolk and her colleagues said this was the first time the potential benefits of fatty fish versus lean fish were specifically examined. Previous studies had analyzed total fish consumption, not taking into account the differences between lean and fatty fish in the content of omega-3 fatty acids and vitamin D.

Though the results are extremely encouraging, the researchers cautioned that further study is needed, as this is the first epidemiological study addressing the issue.

To learn more: *Journal of the American Medical Association*, Sept. 20, 2006; abstract at <jama.ama-assn.org/cgi/content/abstract/296/11/1371>.

Oil-packed tuna: Sorry, Charlie?

Q Most of us grew up eating tuna salad; unfortunately, it was made with tuna packed in vegetable oil and with Miracle Whip. I understand that water-packed tuna is better for you and I have been cutting the mayonnaise with yogurt. Still, I have a fondness for tuna in oil; the taste is different. How about the tuna packed with olive or canola oil? It is a little more expensive and I am sure has added calories, but olive and canola oils are the good fats, so why isn't tuna in olive oil better for you?

A There's no reason not to enjoy tuna salad made this way, advises Tufts' Alice Lichtenstein. "Just balance total calorie intake in other ways. If you make tuna salad with tuna packed in oil, it is unlikely that you need or want to add as much mayo." For comparison, "light" tuna packed in oil has 168 calories in a three-ounce serving, while the same serving of water-packed tuna has just 99 calories. Each tablespoon of Miracle Whip Light adds 37 calories (57 for regular mayo)—you do the math.

Fish: Smoke 'em if you've got 'em?

Q Your newsletter has pointed out the nutritional benefit of eating fish. I am very found of smoked fish, such as sable, chub and smoked whitefish. Do smoked fish have the same nutritional values as broiled, baked or canned fish?

A Smoking fish does change the nutritional value. The other nutritional variable to keep in mind is the variety of fish, as not all species are equally high in the omega-3 fatty acids that have been shown to protect against cardiovascular disease. In most cases, as shown in the chart on this page, fish lose some of these heart-healthy fatty acids in the smoking process. Tufts' Alice Lichtenstein also cautions that smoked fish are relatively high in sodium, which is added as salt in processing. A three-ounce portion of sablefish, for example, goes from 61 milligrams of sodium when broiled or baked to 626 milligrams when commercially smoked. See the chart below for other examples.

Smoked vs. Broiled or Baked

All figures are for a three-ounce portion and are from the USDA Nutrient Data Laboratory.

	Sodium	Total n-3 fatty acids
Broiled/baked Chinook salmon	51 mg	1.728 g
Smoked Chinook salmon	666 mg	0.445 g
Broiled/baked sturgeon	59 mg	0.362 g
Smoked sturgeon	628 mg	0.176 g
Broiled/baked whitefish	55 mg	1.548 g
Smoked whitefish	866 mg	0.178 g

Q At our local supermarkets a fish called "steelhead trout" is sold. The flesh is pinkish like salmon, not like trout. What exactly is this fish and is it a good source of omega-3?

A Steelhead trout *(Oncorhynchus mykiss)* is a rainbow trout that has spent part of its life in the sea. Also called "salmon trout" or "sea-run trout," it's a large, bluish fish that's prized by sport fishermen. According to the Alaska Department of Fish and Game, "There are no major physical differences between rainbow and steelhead trout; however, the nature of their differing lifestyles has resulted in subtle differences in color, shape and general appearance." All trout and salmon, along with chars, belong to the family Salmonidae, sometimes referred to as "salmonids." Steelhead trout are actually similar to some Pacific salmon in their ecological needs and life cycles: Both are born in freshwater streams, then swim to the ocean after one to three years; like salmon, steelhead return to their native streams to spawn, but they don't necessarily die after spawning, as salmon do.

Wild steelhead trout, like wild salmon, get the pinkish-orange color of their flesh from crustaceans and other colorful prey they consume. Farm-raised salmonids are naturally gray-fleshed; producers dye the flesh to make it look more appealing to consumers. Most steelhead trout available in supermarkets is farm-raised.

A 100-gram serving (about 3.5 ounces) of farm-raised steelhead, cooked by dry heat, provides 1.236 grams of omega-3 fatty acids. A similar portion of farm-raised Atlantic salmon contains 2.26 grams of omega-3s. Steelhead trout is high in protein (24.2 grams in 100 grams) and relatively low in calories (170), and is also a good source of niacin, vitamin B12, pantothenic acid and selenium.

Nutrition for Your Whole Body

Beyond Brown Rice: 10 Whole Grains to Discover for Your Diet

As a reader of this newsletter, you already know that whole grains are good for you. But if you're like most Americans, beyond oatmeal for breakfast, whole-wheat bread for your lunchtime sandwich and an occasional foray into cooking brown rice as a dinner side dish, you find it hard to work whole grains into your diet. The latest federal dietary guidelines tell us to "make half your grains whole," but surveys show that 80% of us eat less than one serving of whole grains per day.

To be considered "whole," a grain must retain all of its layers—the fiber-rich outer bran, the endosperm and the nutrient-dense inner germ. When grains are "refined," everything gets removed except the middle endosperm layer. While lots of nutrients get lost in the process, the no-longer-whole grains generally become faster and more convenient to cook—like the difference between brown and white rice.

In fact, however, whole-grain cooking can *save* time in the kitchen. Most grains, even the more "exotic" ones, cook up in an hour or less with nothing more than an occasional stir of the pot from start to finish. A few cook in as little as 15 minutes. Cook up a pot, remove the serving you will consume immediately, and as soon as the pot is cool enough to touch, put the remainder into a storage container and refrigerate immediately. Most grains will remain fresh for a week with this method. Use the leftovers in subsequent meals by scooping out what you need and adding vegetables and/or meats for new and interesting meals with a nutritious whole-grain base.

For even more convenience, put the leftover cooked grain in serving-size freezer bags or containers. When you're ready to use, thaw the grain in a microwave or place the sealed container in cold water for 15 minutes, then reheat.

With a little know-how, you'll discover a wealth of whole-grain goodness in nutritious foods that can take your diet beyond brown rice and whole-wheat bread.

Amaranth is actually not a grain, but the extremely nutritious seed of an herb. It was a dietary staple of the pre-Columbian Aztecs in the 15th century. Extremely high in protein, amaranth is a good source for vitamin C and beta-carotene, and has a pleasant, nutty flavor. Amaranth can be cooked as a cereal, ground into flour, popped like popcorn, sprouted or toasted. The seeds can be cooked with other whole grains, added to stir-fry or added to soups and stews as a nutrient-dense thickening agent.

Cooking: Add amaranth to twice as much water for a rice-like texture or two to three times as much water for cereal consistency. Cook until tender, about 18-20 minutes.

Barley was a favorite grain with ancient civilizations, and today is the fourth most widely grown grain in the world. Barley is high in gluten, making it excellent for use in soups and stews, and for grinding into flour. The flavor is sweet and nutty. High in protein, niacin, folic acid, calcium and other minerals, barley is a good substitute for rice and millet in recipes. Barley is unusual among grains in that its fiber is spread throughout the endosperm as well as in the bran. So even heavily "pearled" barley—processed to cook faster—is full of healthy fiber. And the National Barley Foods Council considers "lightly pearled" barley synonomous with "hulled" barley, the term for minimally processed barley. You'll also see terms like "Pot" or "Scotch" barley. For maximum whole-grain goodness, seek out "hulled" barley in your local natural-foods store—but any barley is good for you.

Cooking: Boil four cups of water and add one cup of barley; reduce heat, cover and cook one hour. Yields four cups. Barley cooked this way can be served as a savory or sweet side dish—with added vegetables, or with dried fruit, nuts, honey and grated orange rind.

Buckwheat, despite its name, has nothing to do with wheat and is, in fact, gluten-free. The seed of an herb, buckwheat comes originally from Russia. It is sometimes referred to as "groats" (hulled, crushed kernels) or "kasha" (roasted). Whole-grain buckwheat may be used as a main or side dish, or added to casseroles or soups. Buckwheat flour, which is robust, dark and slightly sweet, makes hearty pancakes, waffles, muffins and breads. It is best used in combination with lighter flours when baking. Buckwheat contains the bioflavonoid rutin, folic acid and vitamin B6, calcium and iron and is high in protein.

Cooking: Use about two cups water per one cup buckwheat groats. Bring to a boil, reduce heat, and simmer 20-30 minutes or until tender and no longer crunchy (adding extra water, if needed). For a main dish or side dish, try cooking onions with the buckwheat, and add herbs and sea salt during the last 10 minutes of cooking time. For kasha (toasted buckwheat), place one cup in a skillet over medium-high heat and stir in a beaten egg; stir constantly until each grain is separate and dry. Add two cups boiling water or stock, reduce heat, cover tightly and cook 30 minutes. Serve with a little butter, if desired.

Exotic Options

More "exotic" whole grains to consider:

KAMUT: An unhybridized strain of wheat, originally cultivated in Egypt during the time of the pharaohs. Many people allergic to common wheat can tolerate kamut without any reaction. It is highly digestible and rich in protein. Use kamut flour in place of common wheat flour in most recipes. Rolled kamut (like rolled oats) makes a great cereal and is available in natural-foods stores. In addition to protein, kamut contains pantothenic acid, calcium, magnesium, phosphorous, potassium and zinc.

SPELT: An ancient cereal grain native to southern Europe. It is an excellent high-gluten substitute for those allergic to wheat, and can be substituted for wheat in most recipes. It can be found in berry, rolled and flour forms. Spelt is easier to digest than most grains, and is higher in balanced amino acids, fats and crude fiber than common wheat. Spelt contains a good dose of protein, the B vitamins riboflavin, niacin and thiamin, and the minerals iron and potassium.

TRITICALE: A nutritious hybrid of wheat and rye that is higher in fiber than wheat, and contains more protein than either of its parents. Triticale may be found in whole berry form, rolled like oats, or pre-ground into flour. The berries or rolled triticale can be used as cereal, in casseroles or in side dishes. Triticale delivers a good dose of niacin and iron, as well as calcium and vitamin E.

Millet is a protein-rich cereal grass, and a dietary staple in many regions of Asia and Africa. Centuries before corn was introduced to northern Italy, millet was the dietary staple and, in all likelihood, was the original base for polenta. Millet may be prepared like rice and used for hot cereal or pilaf, served with spices and flavorings as a main or side dish, or can simply be added to soups and casseroles or ground into flour. In addition to protein, millet provides calcium, iron, magnesium, potassium and phosphorous. Since it is bland tasting, millet is best used in combination with stronger flavors, as it is in many African dishes that include dried fruits, cinnamon and nutmeg, or Persian recipes that flavor with garlic and mint.

Cooking: For hot cereal, roast uncooked millet in a dry pan for a few minutes; bring two cups of water to a boil, add 1/2 cup millet, and return to boil. Reduce heat, cover, and simmer about 20-30 minutes. Add raisins or chopped dates (optional) during last 10 minutes of cooking time and serve thinned to desired consistency with low-fat milk or fruit juice, sweetened with a little honey or maple syrup, if desired. For other uses, such as main dish or to add to breads, reduce water to 1-1/2 cups.

---

3 Familiar Choices
And don't forget whole-grain versions of these old favorites!

CORN: Whole sweet corn may be cut from the cob and added to soups, casseroles, breads, salsa and more. Cornmeal and corn flour are low in gluten. Corn supplies protein, lysine, vitamin A, folic acid, potassium, calcium, phosphorous and potassium.

RICE: In short, medium and long-grain varieties, whole-grain "brown" rices are generous in B vitamins and E and some–like basmati–are also high in protein. Wild rice is actually the seed of a wild grass, and also is extremely nutritious.

WHEAT: Unlike white flour, whole-wheat flour still contains the germ and bran rich in the B vitamins and E, and has not been treated with bleaching chemicals. Stone-ground flours are preferable. Wheat berries can be soaked and cooked up for an interesting side dish. Besides B-complex and vitamin E, wheat provides protein, calcium, iron, magnesium, phosphorous and potassium.

Oats are a wonderfully nutritious grain that deserve discovering beyond their "instant" incarnations. They provide a healthy serving of cholesterol-lowering fiber and are abundant in protein, calcium, iron, potassium, vitamin A, thiamin and pantothenic acid. When steamed and flattened, whole oats (groats) become "rolled" oats (aka "old-fashioned" oats or oatmeal). Steel-cut oats, or "Scotch" oats, are made from groats that have been cut into pieces but not steamed and rolled. Oat flour is made from ground groats, and oat bran is the outer layer of whole oats, adding fiber but not many of the other nutrients of the whole grain.

Cooking: For cereal, pour 1/2 cup rolled oats slowly into one cup boiling water. Reduce heat, cover, and simmer for 15 minutes, stirring occasionally and adding more water if necessary. Serve with low-fat milk and sweeten, if desired. Groats may also be prepared like rice for an interesting side dish: Toast in a saucepan over medium heat for about four minutes, until groats are aromatic and a shade darker. Add 1-3/4 cups water or stock and a tablespoon of olive oil and bring to a boil. Flavor with herbs, spices and vegetables as desired. Lower heat and simmer, covered, for 45 minutes or until liquid is dissolved.

Quinoa, pronounced "KEEN-wah," is a highly nutritious, gluten-free, protein-rich "super-grain" that (again) is not actually a grain. This tiny seed is a nutritional powerhouse, containing all eight essential amino acids. Quinoa originated centuries ago in South America and is now cultivated in North America's Rocky Mountains. Higher in unsaturated fats and lower in carbohydrates than most grains, it is lighter than rice and can be used in place of rice in cereals, main dishes, soups, side dishes, salads and desserts. And quinoa cooks in half the time of rice. In addition to its protein punch, quinoa contains calcium, iron, phosphorous, vitamin E and lysine.

Cooking: Rinse thoroughly by rubbing grains together in water in order to remove the bitter-tasting saponin, a sticky substance on the outer part of quinoa that naturally repels birds and insects. Bring two to three cups water to boil and add one cup quinoa; reduce heat and simmer until tender.

Rye was popular in medieval times throughout northern Europe and the area now known as Russia. Rye can be found in whole grain, flour, grits or meal forms. Use whole rye flour in making heavy, dark breads and pancakes, or soak and steam rye berries for a nutritious and interesting side salad. Rye provides more lysine than any other grain, as well as protein, calcium, magnesium and potassium.

Cooking: Presoak 1 cup whole rye in 2-1/2 cups water overnight. Change water, bring to boil, and simmer 45-60 minutes, until tender. Add vegetables and drizzle with low-fat salad dressing.

To learn more: Whole Grains Council, <www.wholegrainscouncil.org>.

FDA OKs Barley Claim, Nixes Whole-Grains Labels

If you're confused about the health claims made by various grain products, you're not alone. And two recent rulings from the US Food and Drug Administration (FDA)—one of them aimed at *preventing* consumer confusion—may leave you scratching your head even more.

On the one hand, the FDA approved a health claim for barley, allowing products to state that its beta-glucan soluble fiber may reduce the risk of heart disease. On the other hand, the FDA rejected a General Mills petition asking for labels differentiating sources of whole grain based on fiber content.

FDA Defines "Whole Grains"

Confused about what is and isn't a "whole grain," and how to get enough in your diet? The US Food and Drug Administration (FDA) hopes to help, issuing its first official definition of "whole-grain foods." Although the draft guidelines were created for food packagers, FDA officials also stressed the importance to consumers of consistent and uniform terminology.

The new FDA guideline defines a "whole-grain food" as containing all three ingredients of a cereal grain—the outer bran, the inner endosperm and the germ—in the same relative proportion as found in nature. Typically, the endosperm is all that's left after grains have been processed, whereas whole grains also retain the fiber-rich bran and healthful germ. By requiring food companies to stick to a grain's natural proportions, the FDA aims to keep them from adding back a smidgen of bran and germ to processed grains and labeling the result "whole."

"Whole grains," according to the FDA, may include barley, buckwheat, bulgur, corn, millet, rice, rye, oats, sorghum, wheat and wild rice. Although rolled and "quick oats" can continue to be called "whole grains" because they contain all of their bran, germ and endosperm, other widely used food products may not meet the new definition. Products the FDA does not consider "whole grains" include those derived from legumes (soybeans), oilseeds (sunflower seeds) and roots (arrowroot).

To learn more: FDA <www.fda.gov/bbs/topics/ news/2006/NEW01317.html>.

The barley ruling, at least, is straightforward: The FDA cited five clinical trials testing the effect of consuming whole-grain barley and dry milled barley products that consistently reported reductions in total and LDL ("bad") cholesterol. Although the cholesterol drops weren't huge—one 2004 study found a 6-8% LDL improvement—the FDA said the barley benefits were statistically significant.

Products eligible for the health claim include whole grain barley, barley bran, barley flakes, barley grits, barley flour, barley meal and pearl barley. To qualify, a product must contain at least 0.75 grams of beta-glucan soluble fiber per serving. Unlike many other grains, beta-glucan soluble fiber is found throughout the barley kernel, not just in the outer bran layer that's typically lost in processing.

Expect to find health claims like this on barley products: "Soluble fiber from foods such as [name of food], as part of a diet low in saturated fat and cholesterol, may reduce the risk of heart disease. A serving of [name of food] supplies [x] grams of the soluble fiber necessary per day to have this effect." The claim is based on consuming a total of three grams of the fiber daily.

The whole-grains ruling is a bit more complicated. General Mills asked the FDA to approve three different labels for whole-grain foods, based on fiber per serving: "excellent source" of whole grain (16 grams or more of fiber), "good source" (8-15 grams) and "made with whole grain" (at least 8 grams). The FDA refused, stating that the terms "excellent source" and "good source" have been defined for use only with nutrients that have an established reference daily basis (RDI) or daily reference value (DRV). The latest federal dietary guidelines recommend increased consumption of whole grains, at least three servings per day. But there is no established RDI or DRV for whole grains.

Moreover, the FDA noted that scientific evidence suggests the health benefits of whole grains are based on more than just fiber content. So a labeling system measuring only fiber would confuse consumers instead of guiding them.

Until this all gets sorted out, make sure the first item on a product's list of ingredients is a whole grain, such as "whole wheat." You can also look for the Whole Grain Stamp, introduced in January 2005 by the Whole Grains Council.

To learn more: National Barley Foods Council <www.barleyfoods.org>.
Whole Grains Council <www.wholegrainscouncil.org>.

Add Lower Diabetes Risk to Benefits from Low-Fat Dairy

Ladies, raise your glasses—of low-fat milk, that is. There's even more good news about low-fat dairy and women's health. A new study suggests that a diet rich in low-fat dairy products may lower the risk of type 2 diabetes in women, mirroring the positive findings of an earlier study that showed similar benefits in men.The study, published in *Diabetes Care*, looked for the relationship between type 2 diabetes and consumption of dairy foods in 37,183 women participating in the Women's Health Study. Over 10 years, 1,603 women in the group developed diabetes.

After adjusting for potentially confounding factors—such as weight, physical activity and family history of diabetes—women with the highest intake of low-fat dairy foods were shown to be 21% less likely to develop type 2 diabetes than those with the lowest intake. In fact, each additional daily serving of low-fat dairy was associated with a 4% lower risk of developing type 2 diabetes.

The benefit of the high intake of low-fat dairy foods was independent of dietary calcium and vitamin D. This was the first study in which the effects of those nutrients were "teased out" of the results to specifically consider the benefits of dairy consumption and type 2 diabetes risk, the study's authors said.

"The most important finding is that women who consumed more low-fat dairy foods tended to experience a lower risk of type 2 diabetes in a period of 10 years," Simin Liu, MD, ScD, professor of epidemiology at UCLA School of Public Health and lead author of the study, told Reuters Health. "The message is that low-fat dairy foods can be incorporated into a healthy diet that may lower a woman's risk of diabetes."

Other recent studies have suggested that increased consumption of low-fat dairy products may enhance weight loss, lower blood pressure and lower the risk of developing insulin resistance syndrome, a precursor to type 2 diabetes. But studies examining the link between these factors and diabetes risk have been sparse, prompting their research, the authors said.

While the findings are promising, Dr. Liu and his colleagues caution that further research is needed to confirm their observations before wide-scale recommendations to increase dairy consumption for lower risk of type 2 diabetes.

To learn more: *Diabetes Care*, July 2006; abstract at
<care.diabetesjournals.org/ cgi/content/abstract/29/7/1579>.

Vegetables May Help Prevent Diabetes– Unless You Smoke

Chomping a few extra carrots may help you ward off diabetes—if you don't smoke. Smoking, however, seems to nullify the protective effects of high levels of carotenoids. Naturally occurring antioxidant pigments that give carrots and tomatoes their orange-red color, carotenoids are also found in dark leafy greens such as spinach and kale.

Previous studies have connected high carotenoid levels in the blood with reduced diabetes risk, and linked smoking with low carotenoid levels. A team of researchers, led by David R. Jacobs, Jr., MD, of the University of Minnesota School of Public Health, sought to put these connections together: Would the rare smoker with high carotenoid levels still enjoy a reduced diabetes risk?

Their conclusion was no, that smoking somehow blocks the protective benefits of carotenoids.

The researchers analyzed data from 4,493 participants, ages 18 to 30, in the Coronary Artery Risk Development in Young Adults study. During 16 years of followup, 148 of that group developed diabetes. Nonsmokers with high carotenoid levels were less likely to develop diabetes, but smokers saw no similar benefit.

Carotenoids may counteract oxidative stress in the body, the researchers speculated, thereby reducing a person's risk of developing diabetes. But this "antioxidant metabolism and the oxidative defense system behave differently in smokers than in nonsmokers."

So, if you want to add to your armor against diabetes, remember to eat your vegetables, especially brightly colored veggies and dark leafy greens. But if you smoke, it seems that all the carrots in the world won't help you beat diabetes—unless you quit.

To learn more: *American Journal of Epidemiology*, May 15, 2006; abstract at <aje.oxfordjournals.org/ cgi/content/abstract/163/10/929>.

Magnesium Found to Fight Metabolic Syndrome

A diet rich in magnesium may help reduce the risk of metabolic syndrome and, perhaps, a heart attack or diabetes. That's the conclusion of new research funded by the National Heart, Lung and Blood Institute, and published in the American Heart Association journal *Circulation*.

Previous studies have indicated that magnesium can reduce the risk of individual components of metabolic syndrome. But, according to the lead author of the new study, Ka He, MD, ScD, assistant professor of preventive medicine at Northwestern University, "As far as we can determine, this is the first prospective evidence that shows magnesium intake provides a beneficial effect in the syndrome."

Metabolic syndrome is a cluster of cardiovascular disease and diabetes risk factors including excess waist circumference, high blood pressure, elevated triglycerides, low levels of high-density lipoprotein (HDL, the "good" cholesterol) and high fasting glucose levels. The presence of three or more factors increases your risk of developing diabetes and cardiovascular disease.

The observational study tracked 4,637 men and women, ages 18 to 30, enrolled in the Coronary Artery Risk Development in Young Adults Study. The age of the participants at enrollment was important, Dr. He noted, because "most of the evidence that magnesium lowers the risk of cardiovascular disease or diabetes comes from studies of older adults. People middle-aged or older are more likely to already have the onset of disease."

Fifteen years later, 608 participants had developed metabolic syndrome.

How Magnesium Adds Up

How much magnesium is enough? After age 30, the Institute of Medicine recommends 420 milligrams daily for men and 320 for women. Good dietary sources
of magnesium include halibut, almonds, cashews, spinach, whole-grain cereals,
black-eyed peas, long-grain brown rice, kidney and pinto beans, avocadoes,
bananas and raisins.

The researchers divided the volunteers into four equal-sized groups ("quartiles") based on magnesium intake. Most got their magnesium from dietary
sources; only 16% took dietary supplements containing magnesium.

The researchers found that the more magnesium a person consumed,
the less his or her risk of metabolic syndrome. Compared with those in
the lowest-magnesium group, those with the highest intake had a 31%
reduced risk of developing the syndrome. "We saw a risk reduction for
the upper three quartiles but it was only statistically significant in the
two highest-intake groups," Dr. He said. "We also saw that a higher
magnesium intake was associated with a reduced risk of each individual
component of the metabolic syndrome."

But Dr. He cautioned against relying on magnesium alone to ward off
metabolic syndrome. "Magnesium is just one component of a healthy diet,
and a healthy diet is just one component of a healthy lifestyle," he said. "In
general, people should eat more fruits and vegetables and reduce their
intake of saturated fats and trans fats, get more physical activity, and stop
smoking."

To learn more: *Circulation*, April 4, 2006; abstract online at
<circ.ahajournals.org/cgi/content/abstract/113/13/1675>.

Higher Vitamin D Amounts Linked to Stronger Lungs

Researchers keep discovering new benefits from getting enough vitamin
D, which has been linked to everything from stronger bones to preventing prostate cancer. Now a study, recently published in *Chest*, has
found that the higher the level of vitamin D in your blood, the better your
lungs seem to function.

Researchers at the University of Auckland in New Zealand analyzed
data on 14,091 American adults collected from 1988-1994 as part of the
US National Health and Nutrition Examination Survey (NHANES). They

broke the subjects into five groups, based on serum concentrations of vitamin D, then compared how much air they could exhale in one second (forced expiratory volume, or FEV) as well as forced vital capacity, FVC, the amount a person can blow after a deep breath when exhaling as rapidly as possible.

Even after adjusting for factors such as smoking and exercise, the group with the highest vitamin D levels had substantially stronger FEV scores and better FVC rates. The difference based on vitamin D was greater even than that between subjects who'd never smoked and ex-smokers. The strongest correlation between lung function and vitamin D was found in those who were over the age of 60 and in smokers.

Study lead author Peter N. Black, ChB, cautioned, "Although there is a definite relationship between lung function and vitamin D, it is unclear if increases in vitamin D through supplements or dietary intake will actually improve lung function in patients with chronic respiratory diseases" such as COPD, asthma and emphysema. The researchers speculated that vitamin D may help in the remodeling of tissues in the lung.

In an accompanying editorial, Harvard Medical School professor Rosalind Wright, MD, MPH, expressed hope that vitamin D will eventually be proven to be a "simple, low-cost intervention that would likely have high compliance to prevent of slow loss of lung function in susceptible subgroups."

The study also found more vitamin D naturally in men than in women and less vitamin D the older and more obese a person becomes. Although the body naturally produces vitamin D from sunlight and the vitamin is found in foods such as fortified milk and fatty fish, it's difficult to get enough from natural sources alone, especially during the winter in northern latitudes. The recommended daily dose of vitamin D is 400 international units (IU), though many experts believe older adults need twice that amount, or even 1,000 IU.

To learn more: *Chest*, December 2005; free abstract online at
<www.chestjournal.org/cgi/ content/abstract/128/6/3792>.

Antioxidants in Diet Could Help You Breathe Easier as You Get Older

French researchers have found that dietary beta-carotene could help slow the natural decline in lung function with age. Comparing breathing tests in subjects eight years apart, the study discovered that those with the highest blood levels of beta-carotene—a dietary antioxidant—retained over 20% more lung function than those with the lowest beta-carotene levels. Over a 10-year span, researchers noted, the benefit of a specific increase in beta-carotene levels "approximately counteracts the effect of one year of aging."

The study also found that beta-carotene together with vitamin E, another antioxidant, appeared to protect against decline in lung function due to smoking. Among smokers with a greater than a pack-a-day habit, those with the lowest beta-carotene and vitamin E levels showed double the decline in lung function. Lead author Armelle Guénégou, PhD, of the French national health institute INSERM cautioned, however, that smokers can't avoid the health toll of their habit simply by eating right or taking vitamins.

The researchers began with 1,194 adults, ages 20 to 44, who were enrolled in the European Community Respiratory Health Survey. Complete data was available for comparison on 535 subjects, 40% of them lifelong nonsmokers, eight years later. The subjects' lung function was tested by measuring forced expiratory volume at one minute (FEV1)—essentially, how much air they could forcefully exhale in a minute after taking as big a breath as possible.

"The results strongly suggest that beta-carotene protects against the decline in FEV1 over an eight-year period in the general population, and that beta-carotene and vitamin E are protective in heavy smokers," the researchers wrote in *Thorax*.

The average decline in FEV1 was 29.8 milliliters a year. But the third of the subjects with the lowest beta-carotene levels lost an average of 36.5 milliliters a year, while the third with the highest levels saw an average decline of just 28.6 milliliters annually. Overall, men and those who were obese showed the greatest loss of lung power.

The researchers theorized that oxidative stress may contribute to airway obstruction over time, so

> ## On the Other Hand...
> The new French study showing lung benefits for beta-carotene contrasts with another recent French research report. That 10-year study, published last fall in the *Journal of the National Cancer Institute*, warned that a high beta-carotene intake actually doubled the risk of tobacco-related cancers in both current and former smokers. Non-smoking women with high doses of beta-carotene did show a reduced cancer risk, however.

they looked at blood levels of several antioxidants. Only beta-carotene and vitamin E, however, showed benefits in slowing the decline in lung power, not a related compound called alpha-carotene or vitamin A. And vitamin E was protective only in heavy smokers.

While seemingly linked to lung health, beta-carotene alone can't keep your lungs "young," the researchers added. They emphasized the importance of a healthy diet, especially with a mix of antioxidants and other nutrients from colorful plant foods, rather than relying on supplements.

To learn more: *Thorax*, April 2006; free abstract online at
<thorax.hmjjournals.com/cgi/content/ abstract/61/4/320>.

Dietary Antioxidants May Help Fight Macular Degeneration

Eating carrots may actually be good for your eyes—along with other foods high in beta-carotene plus foods rich in vitamins C and E. Those dietary antioxidants and zinc may help delay age-related macular degeneration (AMD), the leading cause of blindness for those age 55 and older, according to a new Dutch study.

Researchers at the Erasmus Medical Center followed more than 4,000 people ages 55 and up for an average of eight years, during which about 13% developed AMD. Based on subjects' responses to a food-frequency questionnaire, those who consumed above-average amounts of dietary beta carotene, zinc and vitamins C and E were 35% less likely to be diagnosed with the disease.

AMD has previously been linked to oxidative stress, which antioxidants are thought to combat. Although earlier studies have sometimes been conflicting or confusing, some have shown benefits against AMD from antioxidants either in the diet or from supplements. In 2001, a random, placebo-controlled study sponsored by the National Eye Institute, the Age-Related Eye Disease Study (AREDS), showed that high levels of beta-carotene, zinc and vitamin C and E supplements reduced by 25% the five-year progression of patients diagnosed with early AMD.

This latest study focused strictly on dietary sources, and actually factored out participants who took supplements. High levels of vitamin E have been linked to possible health concerns (see the January 2005 *Healthletter*), but the dietary vitamin E intake in the Dutch study was well below those levels.

Besides carrots, good dietary sources of beta-carotene include sweet potatoes and dark leafy greens such as spinach and kale. Vitamin C is found in citrus fruits as well as many vegetables such as sweet peppers, and vitamin E is found in vegetable oils, nuts, green leafy vegetables and fortified cereals. Sources of zinc include red meat, poultry, beans, nuts, certain seafood, whole grains, fortified cereals and dairy products.

To learn more: *Journal of the American Medical Association*, Dec. 28, 2005. Free abstract at
<jama. ama-assn.org/cgi/content/abstract/294/24/3101>. National Eye Institute <www.nei.nih.gov>.

Risk of Vision Loss Linked to Carbohydrate Quality

Your risk for age-related macular degeneration (AMD)—one of the leading causes of vision loss in older adults—may depend in part upon your diet. Researchers at Tufts' Jean Mayer USDA Human Nutrition Research Center on Aging and their colleagues have recently focused on the role dietary carbohydrates may play in AMD risk. In a new study published in the *American Journal of Clinical Nutrition*, they suggest it's not *how much* carbohydrates you eat but rather *which* you choose.

Allen Taylor, PhD, director of the Laboratory for Nutrition and Vision Research at the center, and colleagues analyzed data from a sub-group of participants in the Nurses' Health Study. The researchers looked at the total amount of carbohydrates consumed over 10 years and at the dietary glycemic index—a measure of the quality of dietary carbohydrates. High-glycemic-index foods such as white bread or French fries are converted more rapidly to blood sugar in the body than are low-glycemic-index foods, such as lentils or yams.

"Women who consumed diets with a relatively high dietary glycemic index had greater risk of developing signs of early age-related macular degeneration when compared with women who consumed diets with a lower dietary glycemic index," says lead author Chung-Jung Chiu, DDS, PhD, a scientist in the Laboratory for Nutrition and Vision Research. High total carbohydrate intake, however, did not significantly increase the risk of AMD.

"In other words, the types of carbohydrates being consumed were more important than the absolute amount," explains Taylor, senior author of the study.

The scientists examined the eyes of more than 500 women between 53 and 73 years of age, looking for changes indicative of early AMD. They also analyzed participants' diets, as reported in questionnaires administered periodically over 10 years preceding the eye exams.

"Dietary glycemic index may be an independent and modifiable risk factor for early AMD," says Taylor. "The likelihood of having abnormalities characteristic of AMD on eye exams more than doubled for women who consumed diets with the highest glycemic index, regardless of other factors already known or suspected to increase the risk of AMD, such as age, high blood pressure, cigarette smoking and obesity."

Prior to the current study, the association between AMD and dietary carbohydrate had not been examined. "We are interested in studying the role of carbohydrates in age-related diseases like AMD," Taylor says, "because evidence suggests that problems with carbohydrate metabolism in normal people, as in diabetics, may cause damaging by-products to accumulate in sensitive tissues and contribute to disease."

But Taylor cautions, "We cannot say, based on these data, whether or not consuming a diet with a high glycemic index *causes* AMD."

To learn more: *American Journal of Clinical Nutrition,* April 2006; abstract at <www.ajcn.org/cgi/content/abstract/83/4/880>.

.

Reality Check: Vitamins and Supplements, Cures and Claims

NIH Expert Panel Says Jury's Still Out on Multivitamins

Most of the 52% of American adults who take multivitamins—at an annual cost of $23 billion—probably assume that solid scientific evidence supports these supplements' health benefits. Not so fast, says a new report issued by a 13-member National Institutes of Health (NIH) expert panel. "The present evidence is insufficient to recommend either for or against the use of multivitamins/minerals by the American public to prevent chronic disease," the 19-page report concludes.

Despite a raft of (often-conflicting) studies suggesting that vitamins in such pills can prevent some diseases and promote health, the evidence for such benefits is "quite thin," according to panel chairman J. Michael McGinnis, MD, MPP, senior scholar at the National Academies' Institute of Medicine. The panel's report noted that "there are few rigorous studies upon which to base clear conclusions and recommendations. Most of these studies do not provide strong evidence for beneficial health-related effects of supplements singly, in pairs, or in combinations of three or more." It called for further research to address the "important gaps in knowledge on the relationship between multivitamin/mineral use and chronic disease prevention in generally healthy adults."

The panel identified only three cases in which the scientific evidence strongly supports a protective benefit:

• Supplementation of beta carotene, vitamins C and E, and zinc to prevent age-related macular degeneration.

• Folic acid taken daily by women of child-bearing age to prevent birth defects.

• Calcium and vitamin D supplementation to reduce the risk of bone fractures in post-menopausal women.

Conversely, the panel found no evidence to recommend beta carotene supplements for the general population, and strong evidence to caution smokers against them. Regular beta-carotene supplementation has been linked to an increase in lung cancer among smokers.

The panel also warned of possible adverse effects from consuming too much of some nutrients: "This can occur not only in individuals consuming high-potency single-nutrient supplements but also in individuals who consume a healthy diet rich in fortified foods and also consume a multi-vitamin/mineral supplement."

Such supplements, the experts also noted, "are virtually unregulated" by the federal government. Their report called on Congress to boost the Food and Drug Administration's resources and authority to oversee dietary supplements.

To learn more: NIH State-of-the-Science Conference Draft Statement <consensus.nih.gov/ 2006/MVMDRAFT051706.pdf>.

Is Your Vitamin K OK? Tufts Researchers Keep Track

You can't pour a glass of orange juice without being aware of vitamin C, and every milk jug boasts of added vitamin D. Vitamins A and E have made plenty of research headlines in recent years. But the vitamin alphabet doesn't end there: Vitamin K, which is a fat-soluble vitamin, is essential in blood clotting and cellular growth. It is also involved in building and maintaining bone mass.

The best-known form of vitamin K, phylloquinone, may also help prevent osteoarthritis. Sarah Booth, PhD, director of the Vitamin K Laboratory at Tuft's Jean Mayer USDA Human Nutrition Research Center on Aging (HNRCA), and colleagues recently collaborated with Tuhina Neogi, MD, a scientist from Boston University School of Medicine, on a study published in *Arthritis & Rheumatism*. The researchers observed that higher blood levels of phylloquinone were associated with lower risk of osteoarthritis in the hand and knee.

Vitamin K is important for:
• Building and maintaining bone mass
• Blood clotting
• Cellular growth
It may also be linked to reduced risk of osteoarthritis and heart disease.

Booth's past research has also suggested that high levels of dietary phylloquinone may be an indicator of lower risk of coronary heart disease, but not stroke, in women. Among participants in the ongoing Nurses' Health Study, those with healthier dietary and lifestyle patterns consumed higher levels of the phylloquinone type of vitamin K and tended to have lower rates of heart attack and death from coronary heart disease.

"Research is continuing to uncover other potential roles for this form of the vitamin," Booth says.

Much of what is known about the content of vitamin K in the US food supply comes from research conducted in the HNRCA's Vitamin K Laboratory. Extensive databases now exist for the food content of the phylloquinone, one type of vitamin K. Synthesized by plants, phylloquinone makes dark green leafy vegetables the richest source of vitamin K in the American diet.

The Many Faces of Vitamin K

Recently, Booth and her colleagues for the first time reported data on the content of the two other major types of dietary vitamin K—menaquinones and dihydrophylloquinone—in more than 500 commonly consumed meats, dairy foods, fast-foods, grains, cereals and baked goods. The research was conducted under the direction of the Agricultural Research Service (ARS), which is the chief scientific research agency of the US Department of Agriculture (USDA).

"We know that meats, dairy foods and many cereals and grain products contain relatively low amounts of phylloquinone," says Booth. "Our analysis of the two other forms of vitamin K in these foods confirms that no single food item in the meat, dairy, cereal or grain categories is a rich dietary source of any form of vitamin K. However, since many meats, dairy foods, grains and cereals are often consumed in large quantities, they may be important contributors to total vitamin K intake."

Of the other forms of vitamin K, Booth says, "We are just beginning to study the potential biological activity of menaquinones and dihydrophylloquinone. As we learn more, quantifying the content of these other forms of vitamin K in foods is important."

Although several types of menaquinones exist, Booth and colleagues specifically measured levels of menaquinone-4 (MK-4). "We found that the meat and dairy foods we analyzed have moderate amounts of MK-4. Some of the foods with the highest levels of MK-4 include chicken, cheddar cheese and egg yolks," says Booth.

"MK-4 is relatively high in brain tissue," she adds, "but its exact functions are not known. In the future, if we identify functions unique to MK-4, the presence of this form of the vitamin in meat and dairy foods may prove to be important."

Making Trans Fat—and Vitamin K

While phylloquinone and menaquinones are found naturally in foods, dihydrophylloquinone is formed only during the processing of plant oils.

Booth explains, "During a commercial food processing technique called hydrogenation, phylloquinone is converted to dihydrophylloquinone. Commercial hydrogenation also results in the formation of trans fats, which are now known as 'bad fats.'"

Previously, Booth was part of a study that revealed that dihydrophylloquinone is detectable in the blood, and that levels go up with increased dietary intake. In the study, men and women with higher blood levels of dihydrophylloquinone also consumed greater amounts of trans fatty acids.

Booth and USDA colleagues have now elaborated on the previous vitamin K research by reporting in the *Journal of Agricultural and Food Chemistry* that dihydrophylloquinone was not detectable in most samples of meat and dairy foods. But it was found in low levels in fast-food items, such as hamburgers, tacos and chicken sandwiches. Booth explains, "We suspect these foods have more phylloquinone and dihydrophylloquinone than the meats with which they are made because they are cooked in plant oils."

Booth notes, "It is too soon to say if our findings will affect dietary recommendations in the future." She emphasizes that more research is needed to better understand the functions of the different types of vitamin K and which foods contain them, particularly because studies show intricate relationships between vitamin K levels and adverse health conditions affecting large populations.

To learn more: *Arthritis & Rheumatism,* April 2006.
Journal of Agricultural and Food Chemistry, January 2006.

Antibacterial Soaps Don't Beat Plain Soap–But May Risk "Superbugs"

It's cold and flu season, so it's time to break out the antibacterial soap—right? Not so fast, says a group of scientists who testified before the US Food and Drug Administration's Nonprescription Drugs Advisory Committee. Nothing beats plain old soap and water, according to the scientists, and overuse of antibacterial agents risks developing resistant "superbugs."

"There is a lack of evidence that antiseptic soaps provide a benefit beyond plain soap" in healthy households, according to Allison Aiello, PhD, a University of Michigan epidemiologist who led a recent study on antibacterial cleaning products for the Centers for Disease Control (CDC). The year-long study of 224 households found homes using antibacterial soap no healthier than those cleaning with regular soap.

The homes did not show any significant increase in resistant bacteria, but Stuart Levy, MD, a co-author and professor of medicine and molecular biology at Tufts University, says that resistance has already been seen in laboratory studies. Dr. Levy, president of the Alliance for the Prudent Use of Antibiotics, warns, "Bacteria are not going to be destroyed. They've been here, they've seen dinosaurs come and go... so any attempt to sterilize our homes is fraught with failure."

The greatest concern is over the widespread use of chemicals such as triclosan, which can linger in the environment after killing bacteria. Levy's group advocates banning such antibacterials for ordinary household use, reserving them for hospitals and homes with very sick people. Alcohol-based hand sanitizers and cleaners containing bleach are less of an issue.

Regular household soap fights infection by helping to separate bacteria from the skin, so they can be easily washed away. To get the most out of soap, it's important to rub your hands together when washing and to wash for at least 10 seconds.

To learn more: "Antibacterial Cleaning Products and Drug Resistance,"
<www.cdc.gov/ncidod/EID/vol11no10/04-1276.htm>.
Alliance for the Prudent Use of Antibiotics, <www.tufts.edu/med/apua>.

Policosanol, Sugar-Cane Cholesterol Treatment, Proves Not So Sweet

Does policosanol, a mixture of plant alcohols most often derived from sugar cane, really fight unhealthy cholesterol? More than 80 studies appear to prove policosanol's power to reduce levels of LDL, the "bad" cholesterol. Policosanol is sold as a dietary supplement under dozens of brand names, at about $10-$15 for a 60-pill bottle, and is included in Bayer's One-A-Day Cholesterol Plus vitamins.

But a rigorous new German study concludes that policosanol is no more effective against LDL cholesterol than a placebo. And the researchers point out that most of the previous studies of policosanol were conducted by the National Center for Scientific Research in Cuba—a leading sugar-cane producer. Other positive results came from Dalmer Laboratories, a Cuban marketer of policosanol.

The new study, published in the *Journal of the American Medical Association*, was a randomized, double-blind, placebo-controlled trial—the kind of research considered the "gold standard" of scientific testing. It involved 143 people, randomly divided into five treatment groups. Over a 12-week period, each group received a different dosage of policosanol; one group received a dummy pill instead.

According to study author Heiner K. Berthold, MD, PhD, executive secretary of the German Medical Association's drug commission, the policosanol "did nothing—zip." In none of the five groups did LDL cholesterol decrease more than 10%. "No statistically significant difference between policosanol and placebo was observed," the authors conclude, adding that policosanol also failed to show any significant effect in any secondary outcome measures, such as levels of total cholesterol, triglycerides and lipoproteins.

While cautioning that their findings don't rule out the possibility that the "sugar-cane treatment" might be effective in some other formulation or with a particular ethnic group, the researchers noted the lack of any "mechanism of action" to explain policosanol's claimed effects. The product's benefits, they believe, have at best been overstated.

A Bayer spokesperson told the Associated Press that the new study "was not designed to address a claim that along with diet and exercise, policosanol can help maintain healthy cholesterol levels already within the normal range. Bayer makes only the latter claim, and agrees with the authors that consumers should always discuss their cardiovascular risk profile with their doctor."

In marketing its One-A-Day Cholesterol Plus vitamins, Bayer calls its product "the leading complete multivitamin specially formulated with heart-supporting nutrients."

The German study casting doubt on the effectiveness of policosanol comes on the heels of a smaller South African study that similarly found no difference between policosanol and a placebo in a three-month trial of 19 patients with high cholesterol.

To learn more: *Journal of the American Medical Association,* May 17, 2006; abstract at <jama.ama-assn.org/cgi/content/abstract/295/19/2262>.

Saw Palmetto Shows No Benefit for Enlarged Prostate

Can 2.5 million American men be wrong? That's how many are taking saw palmetto extract as a treatment for enlarged prostate, a common condition known as benign prostatic hyperplasia (BPH). Earlier studies had suggested that capsules containing an extract from the olive-size berries of this small palm, native to the southeastern US, might be effective. That helped boost saw palmetto pills to the nation's third highest-selling dietary supplement, behind only garlic pills and echinacea, according to the American Botanical Council.

But a new, federally funded clinical trial found no difference in benefits between saw palmetto extract and a placebo. The study, published in the *New England Journal of Medicine,* followed 225 men age 50 and older, all with a diagnosis of BPH, for a period of a year. A total of 112 men took 160 milligrams of saw palmetto extract twice daily; the other 113 men took a placebo carefully formulated to mimic the extract's strong smell and taste. Researchers theorized that earlier, more positive results in studies of saw palmetto extract may have been due in part to a lack of adequate "blinding"— participants could tell they were getting a placebo.

At study's end, investigators found no significant difference between the saw palmetto group and the placebo group in American Urological Association Symptom Inventory (AUASI) scores, a standard measure of men's urinary tract health. Nor did they see differences in urinary flow or volume, prostate size, quality of life or serum prostate-specific antigen (PSA) levels.

BPH, which is unrelated to prostate cancer, often occurs as men age: The walnut-sized prostate gland enlarges, causing problems with urination as it presses on the tube that carries urine from the bladder.

Many men prefer saw palmetto extract to prescription treatments because of its lower cost and milder side effects. The new study, part of a National Institutes of Health (NIH) effort to test alternative treatments, found no difference in side effects between saw palmetto pills and placebos.

The results shed doubt on the effectiveness of the popular extract, said lead researcher Stephen Bent, MD, of the University of California-San Francisco and the San Francisco VA Medical Center.

In an accompanying editorial in the journal, however, Robert S. DiPaolo, MD, and Ronald A. Morton, MD, of the Robert Wood Johnson Medical School cited previous studies and cautioned that these new results may be due to the lack of standardization in such botanical products. A 2002 analysis of 21 smaller trials involving a total of more than 3,000 men found "mild to moderate" improvement in BPH symptoms from saw palmetto extract.

But Dr. Bent believes these earlier studies may have been skewed by the lack of a plausible placebo for the pungent herb. Previous trials, he adds, were also smaller and of shorter duration, often failing to use the AUASI standard.

The NIH plans a study that will compare saw palmetto with another alternative treatment, an evergreen bark extract called pygeum africanum, as well as with a prescription medication and a placebo. Until those results are in or other trials test a higher dose of saw palmetto extract, Dr. Morton says, "What I tell men is that they may not do themselves any harm by taking saw palmetto extract." These new findings suggest they may not being doing themselves any good, either.

TO LEARN MORE: *New England Journal of Medicine*, Feb. 9, 2006. Free abstract online at <content.nejm.org/cgi/content/abstract/354/6/557>.
National Center for Complementary and Alternative Medicine <nccam.nih.gov>.

Ginseng's Cold-Fighting Benefits May Be Nothing to Sneeze At

Ginseng, long touted as an herbal boost for the immune system, may actually help fight the common cold. In a controlled scientific experiment of a proprietary polysaccharide-based extract derived from North American ginseng, Canadian researchers found a statistically significant benefit.

But the findings, published in the *Canadian Medical Association Journal*, don't necessarily mean you should rush out and buy ginseng at the first sign of sniffles. In an editorial in the same issue, Ronald B. Turner, MD, a professor of pediatrics at the University of Virginia, cautioned, "This is an unexpected result, and the proper way to deal with it is to see what happens when other people try and confirm it. It's premature for the public to take off on this."

The researchers tested 323 subjects, randomly assigning them to take either 200 milligrams of Cold-fX, a commercial ginseng product whose maker funded the study, or a placebo. Both groups were equally likely to develop one cold during the four-month study period, but only 10% in the Cold-fX group caught a repeat cold, compared to 23% in the control group. Cold-fX takers reported milder symptoms, and their colds averaged 8.7 days instead of 11.1 days.

Study co-author Tapan K. Basu, PhD, of the University of Alberta, said the findings can't be generalized to all ginseng formulations. The tested product is a unique formulation composed primarily of polysaccharides, a complex carbohydrate that Basu believes may be key to enhancing the body's defenses.

To learn more: *Canadian Medical Association Journal*, Oct. 25, 2005. Free text at <www.cmaj.ca/cgi/content/full/173/9/1043>.

The sour truth about apple-cider vinegar

Q I have heard that apple-cider vinegar is good for you (and me). Is that so? And if so, how much?

A Mothers-in-law everywhere preach the supposed benefits of apple-cider vinegar, and now the Internet and various shady marketers have joined in claiming that it can cure whatever ails you. In 2003, however, the US Food and Drug Administration (FDA) warned three Internet marketers of apple-cider vinegar in tablet form (so-called "ACV tabs") to cease claiming that their products are effective against ailments including arthritis, osteoporosis, sore throat, infections, high cholesterol, hypertension, laryngitis, nasal congestion, enlarged prostate and even multiple sclerosis. There's no evidence that plain supermarket cider vinegar is any more miraculous. Indeed, the Supreme Court ruling in 1924 that affirmed the government's power to regulate deceptive labeling came in a case regarding apple-cider vinegar.

"ACV tabs" may even cause injury to the esophagus, and at best contain dubious ingredients, if they contain any actual apple-cider vinegar at all. That was the conclusion of a study of eight different tablets published last year in the *Journal of the American Dietetic Association*, which found, "The inconsistency and inaccuracy in labeling, recommended dosages and unsubstantiated health claims make it easy to question the quality of the products."

The minuses of Juice Plus

Q I have a friend who sells "Juice Plus" supplements. The jars claim "blended vegetable juice powders" and "blended fruit juice powders" that offer "whole food nutrition." How safe and effective are these supplements?

A Created by naturopathic practitioner Hubert "Smokey" Santillo and introduced in 1993, Juice Plus is a success story—at least for its inventors—of "multilevel marketing," hitting $6 million in monthly sales by the end of its first year. Whether it's equally successful in meeting its health claims is a matter of debate. Multilevel marketers like Juice Plus' maker National Safety Associates (NSA), Amway and Shaklee rely on a network of distributors like your friend along with personal testimonials to their products' effectiveness. Testimonials, however, do not equal scientific evidence.

Are powdered vegetables and fruits as good for you as the real thing? In a 2005 review in the *Journal of the American Medical Association*, Alice Lichtenstein, DSc, and Robert Russell, MD, of Tufts' Jean Mayer USDA Human Nutrition Research Center on Aging cautioned against popping pills as a replacement for real food: "Nutrient and nutrient-food interactions are complex and have many facets," they noted. Although their focus was on the often-disappointing results from specific nutrient supplements, much the same concern should be weighed before getting your daily produce in capsule form. Juice Plus may deliver the nutrients of fruits and vegetables, but you're missing out on the fiber of the real thing; you're also leaving a gap in your daily diet that's likely to be filled in part with fatty foods. In 2005, the National Advertising Division of the Council of Better Business Bureaus advised NSA to change its advertising to stop implying that Juice Plus Gummies, a chewable pill for children, is a nutritionally comparable alternative to vegetables and fruits.

NSA also makes a number of claims about the disease-fighting benefits of food enzymes in Juice Plus; inventor Santillo is the author of *Food Enzymes: The Missing Link to Radiant Health*. Most people don't need any extra enzymes, and your digestive tract destroys most enzymes consumed in food, anyway.

According to a clinical summary compiled by Memorial Sloan-Kettering Cancer Center, a few small studies have shown that Juice Plus may increase antioxidant levels in the blood and protect lymphocytes in the elderly. But the summary adds, "None of the scientific studies undertaken have sought to prove that Juice Plus is more effective or more bioavailable than other supplements. In addition, no studies exist to compare the physiologic effects of supplementation with Juice Plus and eating whole fresh fruits and vegetables. Juice Plus is distributed through a multi-tiered marketing scheme with exaggerated value and cost."

Does chromium shine vs. diabetes?

Q I just learned that chromium is a glucose-tolerance factor. Would additional chromium help fend off the onset of type 2 diabetes?

A While some studies have suggested that chromium supplementation may lower glucose and insulin levels in patients who already have type-2 diabetes, most experts believe that more research is needed before recommending such treatment. According to the National Center for Complementary and Alternative Medicine (NCCAM), "There is a lack of rigorous basic science studies to explain or support any evidence of benefit. In sum, there is not enough evidence to show that taking chromium supplements is beneficial for diabetes." For those who don't already have type 2 diabetes, in September 2005 the FDA issued a letter stating that chromium (as chromium picolinate) does not reduce the risk of type 2 diabetes or of insulin resistance. Moreover, while short-term use of chromium appears to be safe in the general adult population, even low doses can cause side effects, warns the NCCAM, and "high doses can cause serious side effects."

Research continues, however, to probe possible benefits of chromium. A University of Pennsylvania study on chromium to treat metabolic syndrome recently wrapped up, though results had not been yet published. Yale University researchers are currently studying the effects of chromium on impaired glucose tolerance, which is often a prelude to type 2 diabetes.

Canola oil fears

Q A local specialty-food store was passing out an article about canola oil that says canola oil is an industrial oil, genetically engineered rapeseed, and "deadly for the human body." Should I stop using canola oil?

A The health concerns you cite represent yet another "urban legend." The Urban Legends Reference Page Web site <www.snopes.com/toxins/canola.htm> calls the canola-oil scare "a bit of truth about a product's family history worked into a hysterical screed against the product itself." The canola plant was developed by natural cross-breeding—not genetic engineering—from rapeseed in the early 1970s. As the Canola Council of Canada <www.canola-council.org> explains, "Canola oil is pressed from tiny canola seeds produced by beautiful yellow flowering plants of the Brassica family. Cabbages and cauliflower are also part of the same botanical family. Canola… is NOT rapeseed. Their nutritional profiles are different."

Many of the concerns misattributed to canola oil apply instead to the old rapeseed oil, which had high levels (30%-60%) of erucic acid. Today, erucic acid levels in canola oil range only from 0.5% to 1.0%, in compliance with FDA standards.

The "genetic engineering" of some canola was simply to improve the plants' herbicide tolerance. Canola oil is one of more than 60 bio-engineered products the US Food and Drug Administration has reviewed and approved over the past decade. According to Robert E. Brackett, PhD, director of the FDA's Center for Food Safety and Applied Nutrition, "The FDA is confident that the bioengineered foods on the US market today are as safe as their conventional counterparts." This conclusion, he notes, has been echoed by recent reports by the National Academy of Sciences (NAS), the Government Accountability Office and, most recently, a 2004 report from the NAS's National Research Council and Institute of Medicine.

Keep in mind that all oils are high in calories, but canola oil is among the lowest in saturated fat. It also contains omega-3 fatty acids, which have been shown to lower heart-disease risk, and is high in vitamin E.

Weighing iron supplementation

Q We've heard it might not be wise to take iron. Is there any reason we should not take a supplement that contains 18 milligrams of iron?

A The answer may depend on who you are, according to Richard J. Wood, PhD, policy chief of the Mineral Bioavailability Laboratory at Tufts' Jean Mayer USDA Human Nutrition Research Center on Aging. Dietary iron is essential for important body needs, such as the ongoing need to produce hemoglobin to make red blood cells. Too little iron can eventually lead to the development of iron-deficiency anemia. "If you are a child or a pre-menopausal women, then by all means go right ahead and take the extra iron because you are at a relatively high risk of having low or inadequate iron stores," says Wood. "The iron in the supplement could be of benefit and will do you no harm at this level of intake. However, if you are an adult male or a postmenopausal woman, then you will likely have adequate iron stores already, particularly if you are a male. Older women will not have to face the increase in iron need brought on by pregnancy, so the need to have considerable extra stores of iron on board in the body to meet the needs of a developing fetus is no longer an issue." On the other hand, Wood notes, a number of studies have shown a relationship between elevated serum ferritin, a measure of body iron stores, and the risk of some chronic diseases. But this still remains an area of research controversy. The bottom line? Says Wood, "If your doctor tests you and identifies you as among the small minority of older people with true iron-deficiency anemia, then, of course, you need to be taking much more iron to help fix your problem. But otherwise you probably don't really need the extra supplemental iron. So it is up to you. Will an extra 18 milligrams of iron in a supplement do you any harm? Personally, I doubt it."

Pectin against Cancer?

Q I recently read an article on "Modified Citrus Pectin" (MCP) and its possible effectiveness in fighting cancer. What can you tell me about MCP?

A Pectin is a carbohydrate found in fruit, especially in the peel and pulp of ripe citrus fruits; modified citrus pectin (MCP), also known as fractionated pectin, has been altered to be more easily digested. According to a 2000 monograph in *Alternative Medicine Review*, MCP "is rich in galactoside residues, giving it an affinity for certain types of cancer cells. Metastasis is one of the most life-threatening aspects of cancer and the lack of effective anti-metastatic therapies has prompted research on MCP's effectiveness in blocking metastasis of certain types of cancers, including melanomas, prostate and breast cancers." In 2003, a very small—13 men—study of MCP's effect on prostate cancer did suggest "that MCP may lengthen the prostate-specific-antigen (PSA) doubling time in men with recurrent prostate cancer," in effect potentially slowing the cancer's progression. According to the University of Texas M.D. Anderson Cancer Center, in another study, MCP inhibited metastasis in rats injected with melanoma and human prostate cancer cells. Such animal studies have explored the mechanisms by which MCP works, "but these results have not been translated to humans yet."

The FDA classifies citrus pectin as "Generally Regarded As Safe" (GRAS), and side effects of MCP treatment are rare. It's too early to say, however, whether MCP will ultimately live up to its promise as a weapon against metastasis in humans.

How much folate?

Q What is the recommend daily dose of folate? Is there an upper limit?

A According to the Institute of Medicine, which sets Dietary Reference Intakes (DRI), the recommended daily amount of folate for adult males is 400 micrograms. The recommendation is the same for adult females, except for during pregnancy, when it increases to 600 micrograms daily, and lactation, 500 micrograms. For comparison, a half-cup serving of spinach, a food relatively high in folate, has 29 micrograms. Much of our dietary folate comes from foods that have been supplemented with this nutrient—so, for example, a one-third-cup serving of Kellogg's All Bran Buds contains 403 micrograms of folate, 101% of the recommended daily value.

The Tolerable Upper Intake Level (UL)—the maximum amount of a daily nutrient that's likely to cause no adverse effects—for folate is 1,000 micrograms daily for adult men or women. In the case of folate, the UL applies to synthetic forms obtained from supplements, fortified foods, or a combination of the two.

Focus on eye-supplement overlap

Q I currently take one multivitamin capsule daily. It has been suggested that, in addition, I take another supplement that's designed as a prevention of age-related eye disease. Is it necessary to take both of these vitamin supplements? If I can eliminate one, which should it be?

A While the answer depends on the exact formulation of each supplement, in general a multivitamin should provide most individuals with approximately the recommended intakes of most nutrients, according to Paul F. Jacques, SD, director of the Nutritional Epidemiology Program at Tufts' Jean Mayer USDA Human Nutrition Research Center of Aging. The eye-care supplement will overlap substantially with many of the nutrients in the multivitamin. Some eye products also contain lutein, Jacques notes, but often at levels that are too low to be of much potential benefit: Six milligrams per day has been associated with a reduced risk of macular degeneration, but some eye products have less than one milligram.

For most nutrients the excess intake from taking both supplements may prove unnecessary but will not present any risk. In some cases, however, eye-care supplements have a high dose of zinc. "That might present some risk by itself, but may provide a more substantial risk if the multivitamin supplement also contains zinc—such as a multivitamin/multimineral," says Jacques. The Upper Limit (UL) for zinc is 40 milligrams for adults. Some vision supplements alone exceed this UL—the specific brand this reader is considering has 69.5 milligrams of zinc—and the combined intake from that plus a multivitamin with minerals can be more than double the UL (a total of 84.5 milligrams in this reader's specific case). The National Eye Institute's Aging-Related Eye Disease Study (AREDS) reported some potential adverse effects from the zinc treatment in the study, including excess self-reported anemia, circulatory problems and genitourinary hospitalizations. (See <www.nei.nih.gov/amd> for more on this study.) Jacques cautions, "Individuals consuming such high levels of zinc should be monitored by a physician who is familiar with the potential adverse health effects."

If you're considering taking two potentially overlapping supplements, Jacques advises, compare the total dosage of each nutrient from the combined products to the Upper Limits figures in the Dietary Reference Intakes (DRI) established by the Institute of Medicine. You can find these online at <www.iom.edu/File.aspx?ID=21372>. He adds, "Looking at the content and overlap might also help identify the nutrients missing from the multivitamin and then identify a product or products that augment just those missing nutrients, such as lutein or zinc."

Blood type diet

Q Is there any relationship between blood type and nutrition? Are certain foods detrimental tc some blood types and excellent for other blood types?

A The notion that the four major blood types evolved in different environments and thus predispose people to different nutritional needs was popularized by naturopath Peter D'Adamo in a 1996 bestselling book, *Eat Right 4 Your Type*. According to D'Adamo, people with type-O blood, for instance, evolved as hunters and should eat plenty of red meat, while agrarian type-As should eat more grains. D'Adamo claimed to have collected "over 1,000 scientific articles on blood types and their correlations to disease, biochemistry, nutrition and anthropology."

But a search of two leading nutrition journals, the *Journal of Nutrition* and the *American Journal of Clinical Nutrition*, going back more than 40 years finds only 14 citations even mentioning the words "blood type," none of which have anything to do with matching diet to blood type. A search of the National Library of Medicine's PubMed database for "blood type" and "diet" turns up only seven citations, two of which are articles debunking D'Adamo's theory and none that support this notion. In short, the scientific evidence for this idea is slim to nonexistent.

"The truth is that there is no scientific evidence to support that dietary fad," says José M. Ordovas, PhD, director of the Nutrition and Genomics Laboratory at Tufts' Jean Mayer USDA Human Nutrition Research Center on Aging. "Moreover, I have not seen any serious attempt within the mainstream science to carry out any study to investigate this concept."

Blood type actually has little to do with body chemistry or digestion. And even the classification of four blood types is only part of the story: Since pathologist Karl Landsteiner identified the A, AB, B and O groups early in the 1920s, some 200 different blood group substances have been identified and grouped within 19 different systems.

Most experts discount the idea that your blood type should dictate any departure from the basics of a healthy diet. "Telling people that they should eat more meat because they have type-O blood is irresponsible," argued cardiologist and diet-book author Dean Ornish, MD, when *Eat Right 4 Your Type* was first published. The late Victor Herbert, MD, a physician at Mount Sinai Medical Center and frequent critic of alternative medicine, said the idea of linking blood type and diet is "pure horse manure. It has no relation to reality. The genes for blood type have nothing to do with the genes that handle the food we eat."

Scientists such as those at Tufts' Nutrition and Genomics Laboratory are investigating ways your genetic inheritance might influence your nutritional needs, metabolism, aging and propensity to obesity. But this research looks at genetic factors much more complex than simple blood-type grouping.

Index to topics

A

Abdominal fat—see Belly fat
Acid reflux 48-50
Aerobics 124
Alcohol 34-36,64-65, 72, 85,
    111, 133, 167
Allergies 25
Almonds 45, 75, 82, 156
Alzheimer's disease—see also
    Cognitive decline, Dementia
    52, 126-135
Amaranth 148
Amino acid 68, 92-93, 104 134,
    149, 151
Anemia 174, 176
Antibacterial soap 166-167
Antioxidants 1, 15-16, 19, 25,
    34, 73-75, 101, 111, 113,
    116, 122, 136, 145-155,
    157-159, 172
Apple-cider vinegar/ACV tabs
    170-171
Apples 19, 24-26, 45, 136
Arrhythmia—see also Heart dis-
    ease 142
Arthritis 5, 55, 57, 121-124,
    164, 166, 171
Asthma 157

B

B vitamins (see also niacin,
    riboflavin, thiamine, pan-
    tothenic acid, folic acid)
    68-69, 133-135, 149-150
Bacteria 25, 32-33, 104-105,
    166-167
Bananas 12, 15, 19, 24, 26, 82,
    156

Barley 148, 151-153
Beans 22, 47, 67, 81-82, 86,
    152, 156, 159
Beef 22, 25, 78, 96, 100
Belly fat 57-58, 117
Beta-carotene 16, 148, 157-159,
    163-164
Beta-glucan 151-152
Beverages—see also specific
    beverages 20, 33-36, 43, 45,
    64, 85, 90
Blood type 177-178
Blueberries15, 18, 19,
BMI (Body Mass Index) 37-41,
    43, 49-51, 118, 129
Bone health 15, 71, 81, 123,
    125-128
Bone-density testing 127
BPH (benign prostatic hyperpla-
    sia) 168-169
Bran 19, 147-148, 150, 152
Breakfast 45, 56, 86, 101, 105,
    135, 147
Breast cancer 1, 2, 24, 35, 71,
    106, 114-115, 118-120
Broccoli 16-17, 26, 30, 45
Brown rice 11, 21-22, 63, 147-
    148, 150, 156
Buckwheat 148-149, 152
Butter 47, 86, 95-96, 100, 103,
    107-108, 149

C

Caffeine 34, 36, 47, 72, 90
Calcium10, 20, 31, 35, 42, 91,
    111-112, 114, 123-127, 148-
    151, 154, 162
Calories12, 19-21, 23, 28 30-

32-35
Heart disease—see also
  Cardiovascular disease 3, 10,
  12, 15, 25, 31, 34, 41, 44,
  46-47, 57, 63, 65-70, 72-77,
  79-80, 97, 99, 101-103, 106-
  107, 109, 112, 122, 129-130,
  134, 137, 139, 151, 153,
  164-165, 173
Heartburn—see also Acid
  reflux, GERD 48-50
Hemoglobin 174
Herbal weight-loss 47
Herring 138, 140, 142
High blood pressure/hyperten-
  sion 10, 31, 34, 46, 61, 66,
  71, 79-94, 129-130, 154,
  160, 171
High-fructose corn syrup 18, 35
Hip fractures 125-127
Homocysteine 68-69, 134-135
Hormone Replacement Therapy
  (HRT) 76-77
"Hot flashes" 70-71, 77
Hydrogenated fat—see also
  Trans fat 65, 95-96, 98, 101,
  108
Hypertension—see High blood
  pressure

I
Impaired glucose tolerance 172
Inflammation 122, 134
Iron 9, 20, 27, 29, 31, 42, 149-
  151, 173-174
Isoflavones 70-71

J
Juice 22, 24, 35, 45, 64, 81-82,
  122, 135-136, 150, 164

Juice Plus 171-172

K
Kale 16, 154, 159
Kamut 149
Kasha 148-149
Ketones 47
Kidney cancer 142-143
Kidney stones 82, 125-126

L
LDL cholesterol 67, 70-73, 78,
  95, 97-101, 103-104, 107-
  108, 152, 167-168
Lettuce—see also Salads, Salad
  greens 32-33
Lipoproteins 67, 70, 155, 168
Liquid calories 33-34, 64
Lung cancer 74, 111, 119, 164
Lung function 157, 159
Lutein 101, 117, 176
Lycopene 15-16, 1116-117
Lysine 150-151

M
Mackerel 138-140, 142
Macular degeneration 15, 117,
  159-160, 163, 176
Magnesium 9, 91, 93, 149-151,
  155-156
Mediterranean diet 133-134
Melanoma 174-175
Menopause 70-71, 76-77, 125
Mercury 26, 91, 137-139, 141
Metabolic rate 54
Metabolic syndrome 155-156,
  172
Milk—see also Dairy products
  12, 17, 22, 32, 34-35, 45, 81,
  90-91, 101, 120, 150, 153,

157, 164
Modified Citrus Pectin
(MCP)174-175
Monounsaturated fat 66-67, 87,
106
Multivitamin supplements 68,
164-164, 168, 175-176
Muscle mass 39-40, 53-54
Music 56, 61
MyPyramid 11, 13-14

N
Niacin (Vitamin B3) 9, 145,
148-149
NSAIDs (non-steroid anti-
inflammatory drugs) 136
Nutrition Facts labels 20, 27-
31, 95-96
Nuts—see also specific nuts 19,
67, 81, 148, 159

O
Oatmeal 21, 147, 150
Oats 21, 149-150, 152
Obesity 12, 15, 29, 33, 37, 39-
40, 42-44, 48-51, 61, 64, 93,
117-119, 130, 160, 178
Olive oil 108, 143, 151
Omega-3 fatty acids 64, 101,
133, 13, 140-145, 173
Omega-6 fatty acids 107
Onions 24, 26, 149
Oranges 19, 24, 82
Organic food 23-26, 33
Osteoarthritis—see Arthritis
Osteoporosis34, 71, 76, 125,
127-128, 171
Ovarian cancer 113-114, 116
Overweight 11, 27-40, 44, 48-
51, 57, 61, 106, 119

Oxidative stress 134, 155, 158-
159

P
Palm oil 96, 100
Pancreatic cancer 114-116
Pantothenic acid (Vitamin B5)
145, 149-150
Parathyroid hormone (PTH)
123-124
Pasta 22, 26, 30, 47, 81, 86
PCBs (polychlorinated
biphenyls) 26, 139-140
Peanut butter 21
Peas 16, 22, 26, 47, 86, 156
Pedometers 12, 60
Peel 19, 136, 174
Pesticide 18, 23-26, 97
Phosphorus 9-10, 123
Phylloquinone—see Vitamin K
Phytoalexins 19
Phytonutrients 15
Polyphenols 19, 75, 113, 133,
136
Polyunsaturated fat 102, 106,
108, 133
Popcorn 45, 85, 148
Pork 22, 78
Portion size 28, 30-32, 42-43,
46-48, 50, 63-65, 68, 78
Potassium 10, 12-13, 18, 35,
42, 68, 82, 89, 91, 149-151
Potatoes 16, 19, 25-26, 47, 82,
159
Poultry—see also Chicken 23,
25, 30, 64, 81, 86, 101, 112,
133, 159
Pregnancy 82, 139, 174-175
Prehypertension 66
Prostate cancer 15, 24, 70, 114-

113

Thiamin (Vitamin B1) 9, 149-150

Tilefish 139

Tobacco—see Smoking

Tofu 71

Tomatoes 15, 19, 24, 35, 45, 81-83, 116-117, 154

Trans fat/trans fatty acids—see also Hydrogenated fat 18, 28, 31, 64-65, 94-102, 106-109, 156, 165-166

Treadmill 53, 55-56, 60, 63

Triclosan 167

Triglycerides 67, 70, 155, 168

Triticale 149

Trout 78, 138, 140, 145

Tuna 81, 86, 138-141, 143

V

Vacuuming 54-55

Vegetables—see also specific vegetables 12-16, 19-22, 24-26, 30, 32-33, 42-43, 47, 50,63-65, 67-68, 81-82, 85-87, 89, 92, 97, 100, 105-106, 112-113, 133, 136, 147-148, 151, 155-156, 159, 165, 171-172

Vegetarian 22, 65

Venison 78

Vinegar 86, 170-171

Vitamin A 9, 16, 31, 114, 150, 158

Vitamin B12 68-70, 100, 145

Vitamin B6 10, 42, 68-70, 148

Vitamin C 9, 18, 31, 42, 117, 148, 159, 1163-164

Vitamin D 9, 35, 101, 114-115, 19-120, 123-128, 143, 154,

156-157, 163-164

Vitamin E 3, 9, 101-102, 108, 143, 149-141, 151, 158-159, 163-164

Vitamin K 10, 12, 164-166

W

Waist-to-hip ratio 40-41, 117

Walking 53-54, 57-61, 123, 132

Walnuts 45, 169

Water 18, 22, 26, 29, 32-34, 36, 42-43, 45, 80-82, 86, 143, 148-151, 166

Watermelon 16

Weight loss 2, 4, 27, 29, 38, 44, 48, 53, 58, 61, 154

Weight maintenance 44-48

Wheat 2, 21, 147-150, 153, 153

Whole grains—see also specific grains 11-12, 17, 19, 21-22, 43, 45, 47, 64, 85, 92, 97, 100, 146-153, 16, 159

Wild game 78

Wild rice 150, 152

Y

Yoga 55-57, 127

Yogurt 13, 21-22, 45, 81, 91, 143

Z

Zinc 10, 149, 159, 163, 176

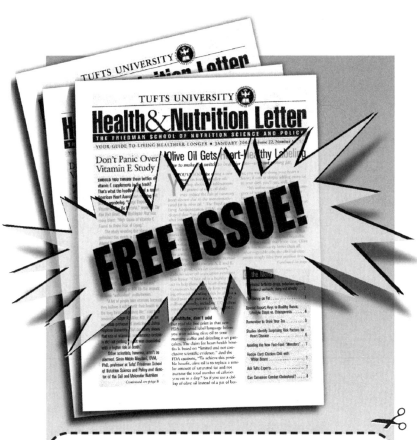

SPECIAL OFFER

✓ **YES**, send me the next issue of the Tufts Health Letter. If I like it, I'll get 9 more issues (a total of 10) for only $15. But if it's not for me, I'll simply return the invoice marked cancel. The free issue is mine to keep. **Guaranteed.**

Name _____ (Please print)

Address _____

City _____ State ____ ZIP ____

Phone _____ Email *(Optional)*

NO NEED TO SEND MONEY, WE'LL BILL YOU LATER!
Canada add $7.50 per subscription. Payable in US funds only.

Mail To: **Tufts Health & Nutrition Letter,**
          P.O. Box 420912, Palm Coast, FL 32142-0912

Or Call: **800-274-7581   (Outside US: 386-447-6336)**

7701HA